Daniel Marchac

Surgery of Basal Cell Carcinoma of the Face

With a Foreword by Claude Dufourmentel

Translated by Eric Pugash

With 80 Figures and 2 Color Plates

Springer-Verlag
Berlin Heidelberg New York
London Paris Tokyo

DANIEL MARCHAC, M. D.
130, rue de la Pompe
75116 Paris, France

Title of the French edition:

Chirurgie des baso de la face – Traitement chirurgical
des épithéliomas baso-cellulaires de la face: Daniel Marchac.

This english edition is published by arrangement with
Editions Médecine et Hygiène, 78 avenue de la Roseraie
Genève, Switzerland

Library of Congress Cataloging-in-Publication Data. Marchac, Daniel. Surgery of basal cell carcinoma of the face. Translation of: Chirurgie des baso de la face. Bibliography: p. Includes index. 1. Face–Cancer–Surgery. 2. Basal cell carcinoma–Surgery. I. Title. [DNLM: 1. Carcinoma, Basal Cell–surgery. 2. Facial Neoplasms–surgery. WE 707 M315c] RD661.5.M3413 1987 616.99'492059
87-26382 ISBN-13: 978-3-642-72813-6 e-ISBN-13: 978-3-642-72811-2
DOI: 10.1007/ 978-3-642-72811-2

Softcover reprint of the hardcover 1st edition 1988

Typesetting: Druckhaus Beltz, Hemsbach/Bergstr.

2124/3130-543210

Foreword to the French Edition

Basal cell carcinoma of the skin presents a very favorable prognostic feature: with extremely rare exceptions it does not give rise to distant metastasis, via either the lymphatic or the hematogenous route. However, locally it has all the features of a malignant tumor: the progressive invasion of neighboring tissues and the inexorable advance of the malignant cells as long as the last one has not been eradicated. This relative benignity is in some respects dangerous, since it encourages overly timid therapy, the more so as one tries to avoid mutilating excisions of lesions located in the face.

The ideal treatment would destroy malignant cells while sparing normal cells. Theoretically, radiotherapy would seem to have this advantage due to the increased radiosensitivity of cancerous cells relative to healthy cells. Unfortunately, this is not the case for several reasons: first, this difference in radiosensitivity is small and one alternates between the risk of leaving residual neoplastic elements and that of injuring normal tissue, especially as the effective dose varies according to the depth of the lesion. In fact, the law of the "distance squared" implies that the amount of delivered radiation and hence its absorption is inversely proportional to the square of the distance between the source and the irradiated tissues. This effect is increased by the degree of "softness" of the radiation which further limits its penetration. Second, it is impossible to determine by clinical examination alone the exact limits and depth of these lesions, and this necessitates the use of stronger and more widely distributed irradiation than is probably required. This results in injury of normal tissues, with sequelae that one had in fact hoped to avoid: aesthetic problems, skin atrophy, dermal fibrosis, telangiectasias, and the risk of subsequent malignant degeneration, substituting a radioinduced cancer for the initial lesion. Finally, the most important disadvantage is that radiotherapy does not allow histologic verification of the completeness of the excision.

Without wanting to deny the value of radiotherapy – a useful method which, in certain cases, should be combined with surgery – it must be said that surgical excision has certain advantages. Furthermore, its disadvantages can be considerably diminished through good technique. Obviously, the principal disadvantage of surgery is mutilation, but technique that is characterized by minimal tension, fine sutures, the use of local or, more rarely, distant tissues, and the concealment of scars in natural folds, minimizes the aesthetic sequelae. The rich vascularity of the face further helps the surgeon to obtain pleasing results. Finally, modern local anaesthesia, supplemented by anxiolytic agents, allows absolutely painless surgery without systemic effects. Generally, surgery can be conducted on an outpatient basis without interfering with normal activities, and requires a minimum of postoperative care.

Daniel Marchac has acquired great experience in the treatment of basal cell carcinoma of the face, not only with primary lesions but also with recurrent tumors and with those operated on elsewhere with poor functional and aesthetic results. In this way he has learned and perfected the techniques and their indications. Moreover, he has understood what not to do and how to prevent those pitiful cases of multiply recurrent and reoperated tumors.

The present work is the fruit of his experience and seems to me to be an excellent update of the surgical treatment of basal cell carcinomas of the face. Although frequently feared by the patient, such surgery presents few inconveniences. The main reason for the still limited use of these techniques is the small number of surgeons capable of applying them.

Thanks to Daniel Marchac, those dermatologists who do skin surgery will be able to widen their activities. Plastic surgeons themselves will find this a guide to improved oncologic as well as aesthetic results. Both will benefit from his teaching.

Professor Claude Dufourmentel
Former Head of Plastic Surgery at the
Hôpital St.-Louis Paris
Member of the Academie de Chirurgie
Member of the Académie Nationale de Médecine

Contents

Introduction

Basal cell carcinoma (BCC) is the most frequent malignant tumor in man (Robins 1975), and represents about 65% of all epithelial tumors (Burg 1975). Cervicofacial lesions account for 93% of BCCs (Pillsbury 1956), and one can say that *BCCs of the face represent approximately 60% of all epithelial tumors.*

The frequency of BCC of the face appears to be rising. These lesions are seen in increasingly young subjects (Marchac 1972), and this is no doubt linked to excessive exposure to the sun's rays. However, this is a "good" cancer since it is localized and easily cured. All treatment methods achieve 5-year cure rates of 95% or more (Albright 1982).

Initially very worried by their diagnosis, patients can most often be reassured about their prognosis. The next question they ask concerns the aesthetic sequelae of the tumor resection. One must ensure the eradication of the tumor, leaving as few visible traces as possible and with minimal inconvenience to the patient.

Surgical treatment appears to be the method of choice in most cases, since it provides the security of resection with fewer complications: surgical excision allows histologic control of the adequacy of resection. The repair is then undertaken immediately, with rapid healing. The aesthetic result is generally excellent, as we will see in detail below.

To achieve a good aesthetic result the repair must be carried out carefully, according to the principles of plastic surgery. Each facial soft-tissue defect poses a particular problem, and ideally, one chooses from an array of procedures the one that will yield the best aesthetic result. This process is best facilitated by plastic surgical training.

Many early lesions are located in areas of tissue excess and can be treated by excision and primary closure of the defect. *These lesions are frequently treated surgically by the dermatologist.*

A study recently carried out by Guiot-Tabernat (1985) confirmed the high incidence of these lesions: 400 surveyed dermatologists saw nearly 20000 BCCs per year, which means 50 cases per dermatologist per year. This study revealed that the majority of the dermatologists treated these BCCs themselves (of the 400 physicians, 220 always treated the lesions themselves, 67 treated the smallest and referred patients with larger ones to a surgeon, 53 always referred their patients to a surgeon, nine treated the lesions themselves or sent the patients to a radiotherapist, while 51 treated their patients themselves or referred them to a surgeon or radiotherapist, depending on the case).

The lesions that them pose the greatest problems are those located on the eyelids and the nose. We will attempt to demonstrate to our dermatologic colleagues how to obtain minimably visible scars. We also think we will be able to show them that to obtain the best aesthetic result after an adequate excision one must often use more complex techniques, in particular the whole range of local flaps. It is obvious that a high degree of technical capacity is required not only to fill a soft-tissue defect, but also to produce the best possible result.

We will describe useful surgical procedures and their application in different areas of the face. They will be illustrated with examples selected from among 650 BCCs of the face treated since 1969. A series of 225 cases with a 3-year follow-up will be presented, along with an analysis of the oncologic and aesthetic results.

We hope that the detailed descriptions that follow will prove helpful to those plastic surgeons who are aware of these techniques but who have not had the opportunity to acquire broad experience in the treatment of skin tumors. We also stress that the surgeon must carry out an adequate excision before concerning himself with the quality of the repair.

Acknowledgements: I would like to thank Professor Claude Dufourmentel, a perfect example of competence and integrity, as well as Dr. Roger Mouly, from whose broad experience I benefitted. They guided my first efforts in the surgery of skin tumors.

I also thank my dermatologist colleagues who placed their confidence in me from the beginning: especially Drs. Paulette Amat, Jeans-Louis Cherif-Cheikh, Hélène Colliard, François Daniel, Victor David, Charles Grupper, Marc Hincky, Jean-Claude Jourdain, Marc Larregue, Chantal Meslay, and France Robin, as well as all those whom I have not mentioned here and who, more recently, have honored me with their confidence.

I thank as well Dr. Claude Demay, who took the trouble to perform the intraoperative microscopic examinations, and Drs. Duport, Lovaas, and Toth, who helped in the analysis of the clinical series.

Chapter 1 Review of Clinical Features and Treatment

As surgeons, we will limit ourselves to the principal clinical features of BCCs of the face, without going into detailed histological descriptions (Casson 1980; Degos 1958; Duperrat 1959; Eade 1974; Pinkus 1966).

In any case, progression is slow and the lesions are painless and cause little alarm, so that a delay of several months to years is usual from the appearence of the first signs until the diagnosis is made.

Epidemiology

Basal cell carcinoma classically first appears in the 50- to 60-year age-group, but in fact we are seeing younger patients with increasing frequency. We recently operated on a 28-year-old woman without any predisposing factors who presented with a BCC of the cheek. As was shown in 1972, in an article entitled "Skin Tumors in Patients Under 40 Years of Age" (Marchac 1972), increasing exposure to the sun certainly plays a large role in the lowering of the average age (61 years for the last 100 patients) of patients affected by these tumors.

Therapeutic irradiation in childhood, such as in the treatment of hemangiomas, is responsible for the appearence of BCCs 10–15 years later, at around 20 years of age. This delay explains the fact that radiotherapists are often not aware of the late complications of such treatment. Even a mild case of radiodermatitis may be complicated by the appearance of a BCC 10–20 years later, especially in the face after exposure to the sun.

It is also not unusual to note a relationship with a traumatic event such as an insect bite or cut. The patient states that the lesion never completely healed or that an indurated scar persisted and underwent progressive change. There may also be a hereditary component, and children of parents with multiple BCCs should be followed up closely. We recently saw just such a 13-year-old child with a BCC of the back.

Clinical Features

The most frequent clinical appearance is that of a raised, pearly pink lesion which is firm, translucid, and well demarcated. Lesions presenting as a chronic ulceration or as a zone of scarring with firm, raised edges are also easily recognizable and well delimited.

The purely ulcerating BCC, or rodent ulcer, is dangerous, since it appears to be limited when in fact it tends to infiltrate widely. The sclerosing BCC or morphea type is particularly difficult to recognize and excise. It often presents as a thickening of the skin, which loses its suppleness and becomes ivory colored. The limits of the lesion are imprecise.

We must also mention the pagetoid BCC, which appears as a superficial pink plaque, and the multicentric BCC.

The size of these lesions is variable and depends on their age and rate of growth. Usually growth is slow, and photographs sometimes show very little progression even over the course of a year. In other cases the lesion may double in size in a few months. It seems to me that the age of the patient is not related to the rate of progression.

Classically, BCCs are located in the centre of the face, predominantly in the nose, eyelids, and cheeks (see Fig. 5.1, p. 85).

These lesions progress at variable rates. Growth remains superficial in certain types (e.g., pagetoid) and is penetrating in others (e.g., evident ulcer). In general, growth is purely local, in continuity, and without danger of metastasis. Nevertheless, the literature contains 130 references to metastasizing BCCs, usually in the setting of recurrent lesions (Baker 1983; Eckhoff 1951; Farmer and Helwig 1980; Koplin and Zarem 1980; Riefkohl et al. 1984; Smith and Irons 1983).

Treatment

Local chemotherapy, in particular using 5-fluorouracil (Heymann 1972), requires prolonged treatment (4 weeks), does not provide histologic control, and may even conceal growth along the deep margin (Mohs 1978). This treatment should be reserved for difficult-to-treat locations in elderly patients.

In situ destruction may be achieved with cryotherapy, radiotherapy, or dermabrasion. These methods appear to be effective and satisfactory results have been published (Albright 1982; Amalric et al. 1974; Kalis et al. 1984; Pierquin 1977). *However, there is no histologic check of the adequacy of tumor destruction.*

Dermabrasion should be considered only for early superficial lesions that do not involve the deep dermis.

Cryosurgery is increasing in popularity owing to improvements in thermal probes and cold generators (Elton 1975; Gage 1975; Kalis et al. 1984). Certain deep dermal structures appear to be spared by the effects of freezing, permitting better healing, and very nice results have been presented (Kalis 1984). However, healing is not always uneventful: inflammatory edema is often marked, especially in the periorbital region; the eschar may remain for several weeks; and hypertrophic scarring as well as hypo- and hyperpigmentation are not rare. Cryosurgery is therefore indicated in the case of multiple lesions and of limited lesions to the alar regions of the nose. It is contraindicated in poorly delimited tumors and in individuals with exaggerated reactions to cold (Kalis et al. 1984; Zacarian 1977).

Contact therapy and electron therapy require numerous treatment sessions (i.e., every 2 days for 4 weeks in the case of contact therapy) (Amalric 1974). The inconvenience is considerable, the adequacy of tumor destruction is unverified, and the complications are not negligible, including loss of the eyelashes following treatment of lesions of the lids.

Interstitial irradiation using 192_{Ir} wire has been facilitated by the use of supple 0.85-mm plastic tubes placed through the affected tissues (Pierquin et al. 1977). The tubes are placed with the patient under neuroleptanesthesia and treatment requires 4–6 days in the hospital. This is usually followed by moderately severe edema.

The difficulty and the cost of interstitial irradiation limit its use to widespread, infiltrating lesions where surgical excision would produce significant deformity, such as amputation of the nasal pyramid.

It must be emphasized that in recurrent lesions following radiotherapy it is difficult to distinguish the tumor from the sequelae of treatment. In our eperience, such recurrences also seem particularly invasive, appearing to assume secondarily the features of sclerosing BBCs.

Finally, it must be remembered that even minimal radiodermatitis may be complicated by the development of a new BCC. We recently saw a 72-year-old woman 4 years following excision of a BCC of the bridge of the nose, who returned with a new lesion of the nasal tip where she had undergone radiotherapy 20 years earlier. This risk must be weighed when one considers the use of radiotherapy in patients younger than 60 years of age (Walther et al. 1981).

Excision without repair by electrocautery has the advantages of simplicity and rapidity and allows a complete histologic examination to assess the adequacy of the excision. On the other hand, healing requires daily dressings for 4–5 weeks to allow granulation, wound contraction, and reepithelialization from the margins. The final quality of the scar may be quite good if the defect is limited and located in an area of skin laxity.

This is a technique frequently employed by dermatologists in their office, but they must be completely familiar with the indications and should avoid using it for widespread, poorly delimited lesions, for those located near an orifice, and for sclerosing tumors.

Mohs' chemosurgery (Macomber et al. 1959; Mohs 1976, 1978a, 1978b) consists of tangential excisions of the lesion with intraoperative histologic examination of each specimen. This technique is time consuming and relatively tedious, and for these reasons is not used in France. However, it provides remarkable security and is especially useful in difficult cases such as those of recurrent, sclerosing, or deeply infiltrating lesions, particularly in the periorbital region. The resulting skin defect is left to heal secondarily. The aesthetic result is often imperfect and necessitates revision surgery.

Excision with the CO_2 laser is a recently developed method which may be used in one of three ways:

1. Simple destruction of the tumor: this has the advantages of rapidity of execution and healing. A critical disadvantage is that the depth of excision cannot be controlled and therefore it is indicated only in very superficial multiple lesions.
2. Excision with laser scalpel and secondary healing: this is a variation of the technique of excision by electrocautery. It provides a specimen for histologic examination and, because it cuts more finely than the cautery wire, allows for more rapid healing and a better scar.
3. Excision with laser scalpel and primary repair: this is a simple variation on the usual surgical technique.

Currettage with electrodesiccation is an imprecise method because it provides no specimen for examination (Kopf and Bart 1977).

Complete, controlled excision with immediate repair is our recommended surgical treatment. It allows (a) complete histologic control; (b) immediate repair, with healing usually occurring in 5–6 days; (c) simple reoperation in case of recurrence, since the limits of the lesion are easily distinguished.

Chapter 2 Principles of Surgical Excision

The surgical excision must be complete along both the lateral and deep margins. The primary concern should be to rid the patient of his tumor by carrying out a wide excision, without considering the repair.

Ideally, the procedure would be undertaken by two operators, the first responsible for the excision and the second for the repair. This is often the case with head and neck cancer, but it is obviously impractical with the great majority of BCCs of the face. Nevertheless, the surgeon should try to separate mentally the excision and the repair, and should never risk an insufficient resection to facilitate the reconstruction. Obviously, this is easier when a variety of techniques are at the surgeon's disposal and when there is always an available alternative in case of unanticipated problems.

For this reason, a thorough preoperative assessment is particularly useful for surgeons whose repertoire is limited, and for dermatologists who are not familiar with all the techniques of plastic surgery. To avoid the risks of imcomplete excision and faulty repair, they must be able to distinguish the lesions that are within their abilities (small tumors in areas of skin laxity) from those requiring the techniques of plastic surgery.

Preoperative Examination

In order for the operator to assess the difficulty of the operation the preoperative examination must include the following:

1. Clinical progression: a slowly growing lesion will probably be less invasive than one that is progressing rapidly.
2. Age of the patient: the excision must be particularly wide in young patients to completely eliminate the risk of recurrence, even though this will make the repair more difficult.
3. Histologic type: sclerosing and ulcerated BCCs necessitate particularly wide excisions similar to recurrent lesions.
4. Tumor location: this can pose problems regarding such adjacent structures as the lacrimal punctum in the eyelids, or such deep structures as the alar cartilages in lesions of the tip of the nose.

An intraoperative histologic examination is planned in difficult cases. It is always indicated in sclerosing and recurrent lesions, and especially those secondary to radiotherapy.

Patient Evaluation

The history must record the use of medications such as anticoagulants, which must be stopped or reduced in consultation with the treating physician. The use of aspirin must be discontinued at least 10 days prior the operation.

Laboratory examinations include screening tests for hemostasis.

There is no known allergy to lidocaine or epinephrine, although there may be hypersensitivity to certain skin disinfectants or adhesive materials. Epinephrine may be contraindicated in certain cardiovascular disorders.

The patient is given a sedative approximately 20 min before the procedure.

Planning the Excision

Under good lighting and 2.5 times loupe magnification, a dotted outline is made of the limits of the lesion using gentian violet ink and a fine brush (Fig. 2.1). The dots are placed along the apparent limits of the lesion including all contour irregularities. The skin is manipulated to test its suppleness, the angle of the lighting is varied, and all suspicious areas are included in the planned excision.

When the limits of the lesion have been identified, the excision line is drawn to allow a 3-mm margin in clearly delimited lesions and a 4- to 5-mm margin when they are less well defined.

A mark is made on the specimen at 12 o'clock to allow the pathologist to orient the specimen. Following excision this point is marked with a suture to ensure visibility (see Fig. 2.6, p. 10).

Preliminary Planning of Repair

Following marking of the tumor it is advisable to formulate a preliminary plan for repair before the tissues have been infiltrated with anesthetic solution. In this way, the skin laxity can be assessed, skin lines can be identified by having the patient smile or grimace, and an accurate drawing of the repair can be made.

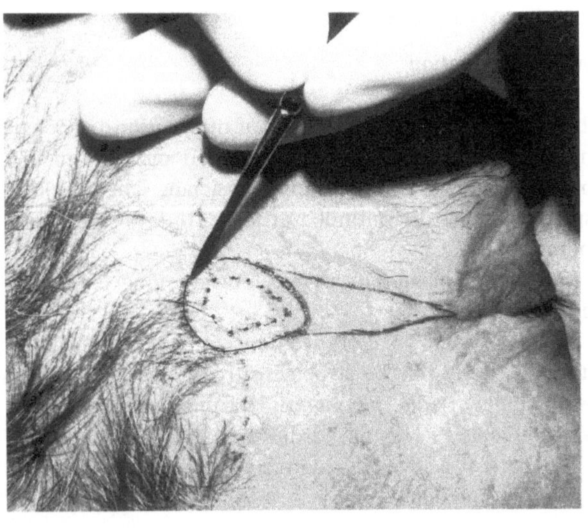

Fig. 2.1. The limits of the lesion are outlined with a fine brush

Local Anesthesia

A fine 0.5-mm needle is used to inject a solution of 1% lidocaine with epinephrine 1:100000. In certain areas one can carry out regional nerve blocks: the infraorbital nerve for the upper lip, the mental nerve for the chin, and the supraorbital nerve for procedures involving the forehead. The needle is advanced to the bone adjacent to the exit of the nerve from its foramen.

In fact, the sensory territories overlap, so that direct infiltration is usually preferable, care being taken to avoid passage of the needle through the tumor and thus dissemination of cancer cells. Infiltration starts at the periphery, along the marked line of excision, and ends at the deep subcutaneous plane. One observes the way the tissues are elevated by the pressure of the anesthetic solution. If the tumor appears bound to the deep tissue planes it is necessary to plan a particularly deep excision.

The Excision

The skin must be placed under tension before the incision is begun. Two skin hooks may be used for this purpose, although I prefer to strech the skin manually with a compress (Fig. 2.2). The incision is made with a disposable no. 15 blade and perpendicular to the skin to avoid bevelling, which can compromise the quality of the final scar (Figs 2.3 and 3.7).

The complete skin incisions is made before the markings are obscured by blood. The incision is begun in dependent areas or where the greatest precision is required (e.g., the medial canthal region) to avoid interference from bleeding.

After the incision has been made, a corner of the specimen is lifted with a skin hook or forceps (Fig. 2.4) and the deep margin is incised. Hemostasis with a cautery is carried out as required.

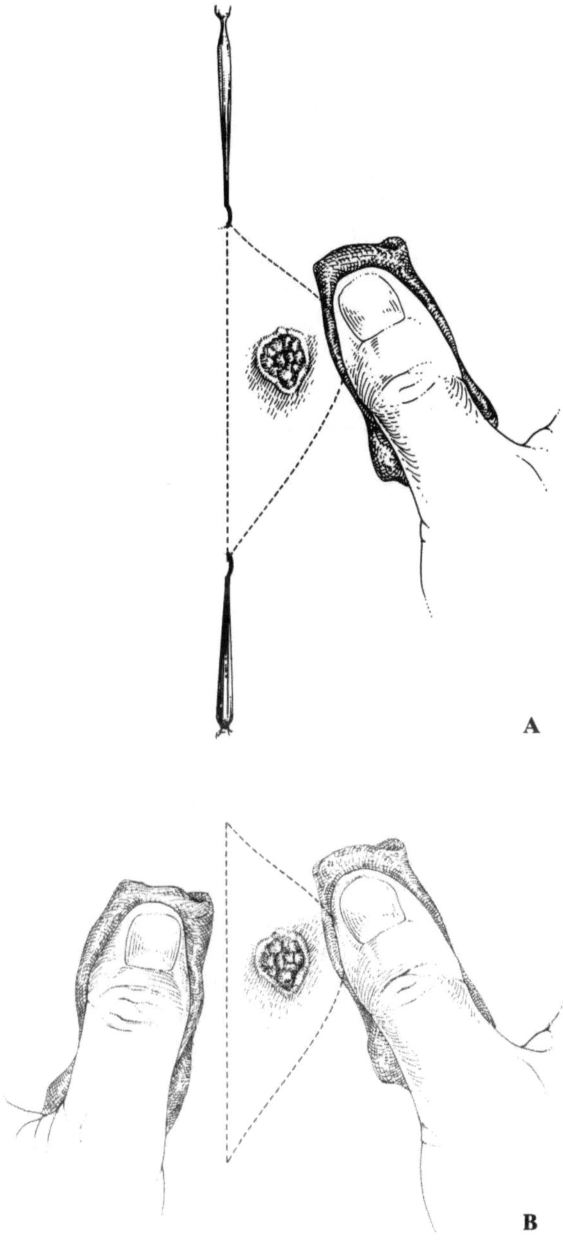

Fig. 2.2. The skin is placed under tension with skin hooks (A) or by pulling laterally on either side (B)

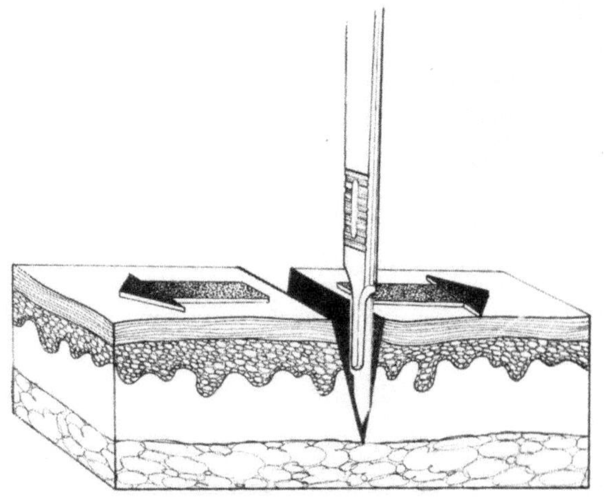

Fig. 2.3. The incision is made perpendicularly with a no. 15 blade

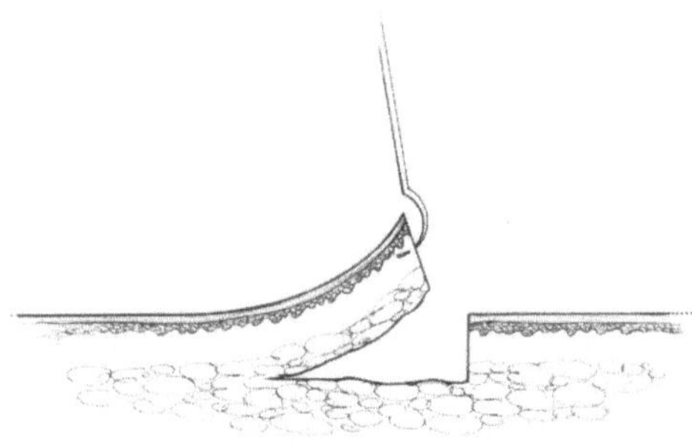

Fig. 2.4. After the incision has been made, the edge is lifted with a skin hook

It is important to visualize the deep plane precisely, and good hemostasis is indispensable. The vasoconstriction provided by the epinephrine is helpful, but bleeding in the face is often substantial. In the nose the skin can be stretched over the pyramid, and in the lips the tissues can be compressed on either side of the lesion. Elsewhere, tension is placed on the skin manually, and the assistant's hand advances progressively to compress the open area (Fig. 2.5).

The deep dissection must leave an adequate margin beneath the tumor. The skin thickness must therefore be

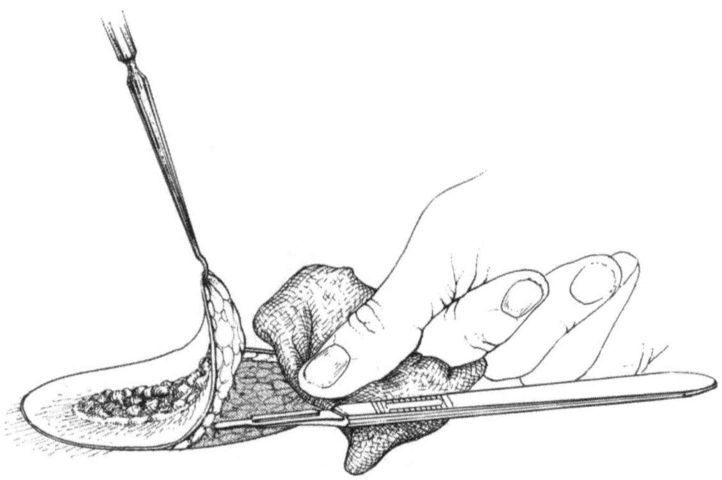

Fig. 2.5. Deep dissection is carried out with a scalpel. The specimen is retracted with a skin hook and the defect is placed under tension and compressed to provide temporary hemostasis

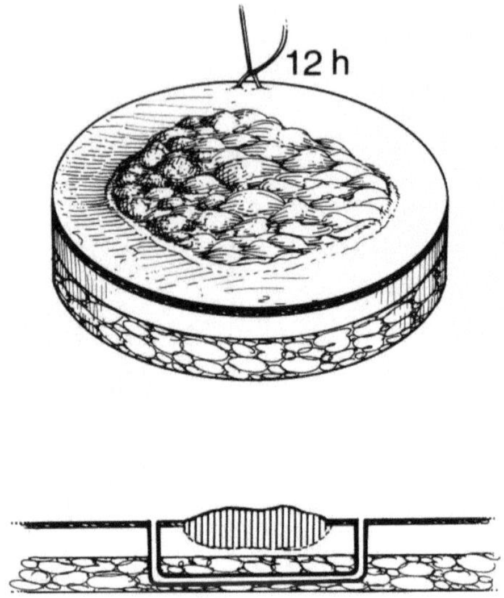

Fig. 2.6. The deep margin is located in the subcutaneous fat. A suture is placed at 12 o'clock to enable the pathologist to orient the specimen

taken into account, as these tumors rarely extend beyond the deep dermis.

If the skin is thick the deep margin passes through the superficial subcutaneous tissue. In the cheek this plane is located in the subcutaneous fat; in the forehead, the deep dissection is at the level of the frontal muscle fascia since the subcutaneous fat layer is thin.

When the skin is thin the deep plane passes through deeper layers. In the eyelids a significant portion of the m. orbicularis is taken with the specimen, since the skin is closely adherent to this structure. At the nasal tip the alar cartilages are nearly always exposed, and often partially removed, to be certain of an adequate deep margin of safety.

After the specimen is removed the deep surface is immediately inspected under loupe magnification. The tumor is sectioned transversely through the centre to verify that the deep margin is separated by several millimeters from the lower pole of the tumor.

The specimen is oriented for the pathologist with a suture placed at 12 o'clock, i.e. at the top. (Fig. 2.6). In the meantime, hemostasis is assured with a fine coagulation forceps (Fig. 2.7).

If loupe inspection or intraoperative histologic examination reveals incomplete tumor removal the excision is extended along the lateral and deep margins. The scalpel blade is changed to prevent seeding of healthy tissues with tumor cells. Repair is not considered before the excision is complete (Abide et al. 1984).

Histologic Verification

Delayed Repair. In certain difficult cases, or when intraoperative histology is not possible, it is prudent to delay repair until the definitive pathological examination has been completed. Repair was delayed in two of the 225

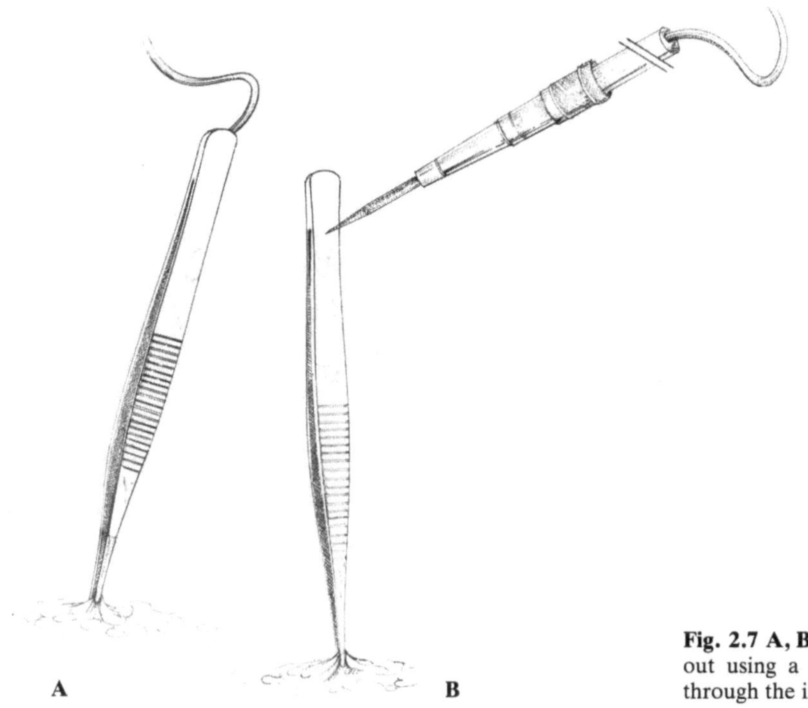

A B

Fig. 2.7 A, B. Hemostasis by electrocoagulation can be carried out using a cautery forceps (**A**) or by passing the current through the instrument that is holding the bleeding vessel (**B**)

cases in the present series. Intraoperative histology is preplanned for sclerosing or recurrent lesions, or for those located in difficult areas. However, unexpected difficulties may be encountered in the operating room, when it is too late to organize such an examination, and in these cases the reconstruction may have to be delayed.

Certain authors, such as Casson (1980), recommend systematic delayed repair to allow time for examination of classical fixed sections. While theoretically safer, this approach significantly complicates the procedure and increases the risk of infection when repair is finally undertaken.

Our series included 193 resections without intraoperative histology, and in four cases the final report indicated an incomplete excision. These four patients were immediately reoperated, and there were no recurrences at 3 years. Therefore, 189 patients benefited from immediate repair, while the outcomes of the remaining four patients were not prejudiced by the necessity to reoperate (see Fig. 5.5, p. 90). It should be emphasized that the specimen must be properly oriented to facilitate later location of the zone of disease, since one cannot rely on the macroscopic appearence.

Intraoperative Histology. This examination is extremely important in difficult cases, but we do not agree with Porte et al. (1979), who advise it in all cases. This increases costs, prolongs the operation, and does not appear justified for the majority of BCCs, which are fortunately well delimited. Moreover, it is not always easy to find a pathologist who is trained in the intraoperative examination of skin tumors and who will take the trouble to come.

Although intraoperative histology is considered to be less reliable than definitive sections, this has not been our experience. In the series of 225 cases analyzed in Chap. 5, intraoperative examinations were used on 32 occasions (by Dr. Claude Demay). The method utilized was the Ultrapack examination technique of Leroux (1931) which takes only a few minutes. The specimen is examined with direct light after staining and thin cuts are not necessary.

There were no false negatives, i.e., in no case was a negative intraoperative exam followed by a report of positive margins on the final sections. None of these 32 cases were recurrent at the 3-year follow-up, although they were by definition the most difficult. Furthermore, in no case did the final section show an unnecessarily wide excision or indicate a diagnosis other than the one of BCC made at the time of surgery.

Of the five tumors that recurred, four were considered to have clear margins on the final sections. In only one was tumor noted near the margins, and this case would probably have benefited from intraoperative histology and a wider excision.

Insufficient Excision. When the final sections indicate an insufficient excision following primary repair, what should be the course of action?

Pascal et al. (1968) studied the prognosis of incompletely excised BCCs and noted that only 33% recurred (14 of 42 cases). They suggest that one can therefore follow these patients closely and reoperate if there is clinical recurrence.

I do not accept this view at all, especially since patient follow-up is not always reliable, and I believe that a 33% recurrence rate is unacceptable. As advocated by Casson (1980), all incompletely excised tumors should be reexcised. This proved necessary in four of 225 cases in our series, and none have recurred.

Borderline Excision. In certain cases the excision is histologically complete, but the margin passes very close to the tumor. Pascal et al. (1968) observed two recurrences in 17 cases of borderline excision (12%).

In the present series four of seven patients with borderline excisions were reoperated on, and they have been free of recurrence. Of the three patients who were followed up, one recurred.

Consequently, I believe that a report of a borderline excision should be followed by reoperation in all cases where the zone of possible recurrence can be precisely localized and the operation is uncomplicated. This is particularly indicated in cases where follow-up is likely to be unreliable, or where anatomically critical areas such as the medial canthus are involved. On the other hand, when the recurrence cannot be localized precisely, when the repair is satisfactory and would be difficult to redo, when the tumor is located in a nondangerous area, and when the patient is elderly and willing to be seen regularly, one may elect to wait. It must be explained to the patient that the recurrence rate is approximately 10%–20%, as compared with less than 2% when excision is complete. In this way the patient participates in the decision and shares responsibility for the follow-up. One must also understand exactly what a particular pathologist means by the terms "limited" or "insufficient" (Abide et al. 1984).

Other histologic features may aid in making the decision whether or not to reoperate. In a series of 57 incomplete or borderline excisions, Dellon (1985) observed 24 recurrences (42%) and noted that the following factors were of prognostic importance:

1. Infiltration of the periphery by tumor cells exceeding 75%, which was associated with a 93% recurrence rate; there were no recurrences when such infiltration was less than 25%
2. Ulceration, which is correlated with a higher recurrence rate
3. Lymphocytic infiltration, which is interpreted as an immune response to the tumor and is associated with fewer recurrences

Although analysis of these features may aid in the decision, the high recurrence rate (42%) at 5 years strongly argues for reoperation in all cases.

Chapter 3 Techniques of Surgical Repair

Basic Principles

The repair should avoid distortion and contour irregularities and be nearly invisible under everyday living conditions. It is essential to avoid excessive tension in order to achieve this result.

When the tumor is located in an area of skin laxity, it is excised elliptically and the wound is carefully sutured following undermining of the edges.

Skin grafts or flaps are required when local skin tension precludes primary closure of the defect. Local flaps provide the best results in the face, and the great variety available makes it possible to adapt to most situations. Full-thickness skin grafts yield variable results and in our opinion are indicated only when a satisfactory flap is not available.

Distant flaps may be indicated in rare cases. These may be either pedicled, requiring section and insetting, or free, with microvascular anastomoses. The slow growth of BCCs may occasionally allow the use of a skin expander.

Closure Is Possible Without Distortion: Elliptical Excision and Suture

This simple method can be used when the defect is small and situated in an area of skin laxity, such as the temporal region.

Design of the Ellipse. Once the excision line has been drawn the ellipse is designed to incorporate the eventual defect.

The ellipse must be carefully planned. The patient is asked to smile or grimace in order that wrinkles and skin lines may be identified (Fig. 3.1). For temporal lesions the patient squints, while the eyebrows are raised for the planning of excisions in the forehead. One must try to foresee and prevent asymmetries in such areas as the nasolabial folds and the eyebrows.

The ellipse should be drawn before the anesthetic is infiltrated, while the skin wrinkles are still visible. It must be made sufficiently long to avoid creating "dog-ears" at the extremities.

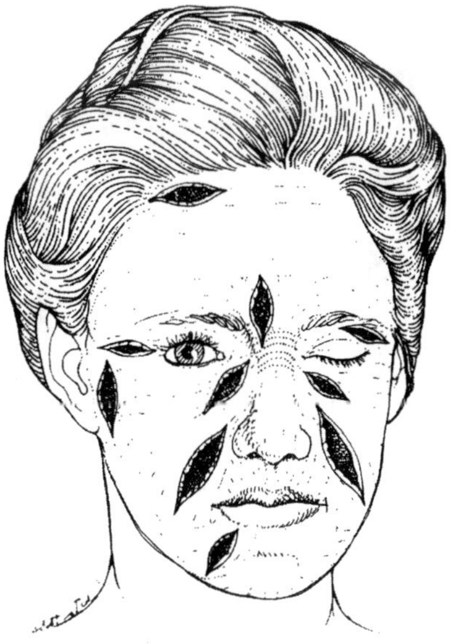

Fig. 3.1. Preferred orientation of elliptical excisions, parallel to the natural expression lines

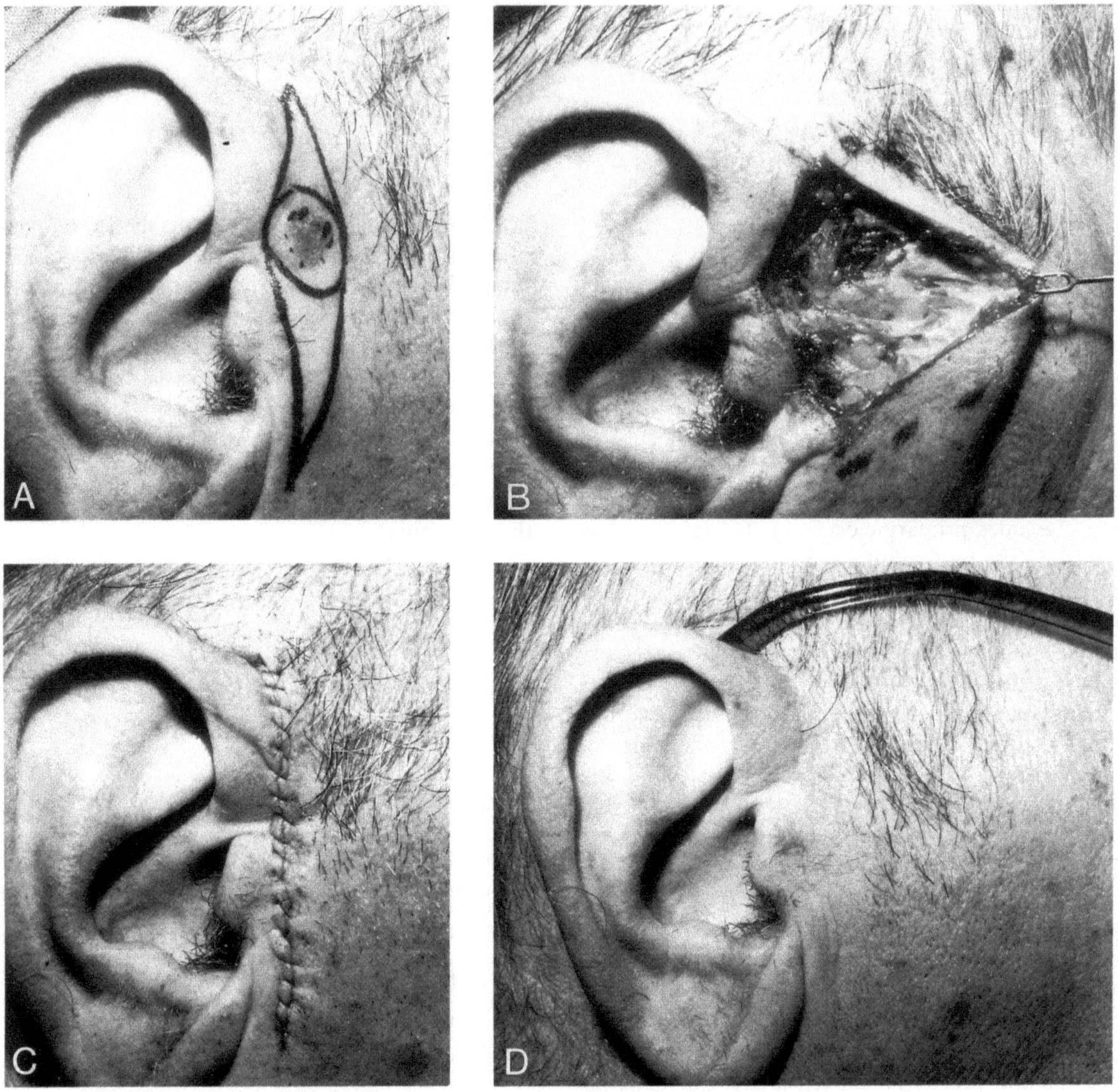

Fig. 3.2. A Elliptical excision of a BCC in a 76-year-old man. **B** Wide undermining is carried out anteriorly to obtain tension-free closure. **C** Closure in two layers with a simple running suture for the skin. **D** Result at 18 months

Except in rare cases, the lesion is removed before the remainder of the ellipse is excised. In this way it is possible to verify that closure will be possible by approximating the edges of the defect.

Excision and Undermining. If the wound will close primarily the two triangles of skin corresponding to the extremities of the ellipse are excised. For the tumor resection (see p. 8) the skin is placed under tension and *strictly perpendicular cuts* are made with a no. 15 blade. Care must be taken to incise cleanly at the junctions of the excision and the triangles of the ellipse. These *lateral triangles* are removed at the same level as the tumor, i.e., in the superficial subcutaneous tissue.

After hemostasis has been achieved, the wound edges are *undermined.* This is critical and allows the margins to be advanced over the deeper planes. This advancement allows good approximation of the dermis and fat to prevent depression of the scar, and decreases the tension on the scar and subsequent widening. This undermining must be adequate (Fig. 3.2), and on each side we extend it over a distance equal to half the length of the ellipse. It is also important to undercut the apices of the ellipse to minimize dog-ears and to facilitate the adjustment of the skin edges (Fig. 3.3).

Undermining is carried out in the subcutaneous plane with a blade or scissors, while the edge of the wound is lifted with a skin hook. It is extended until the margins can be approximated easily. At this point a small amount of fat is removed at each apex to further decrease the risk of dog-ears, and the hemostasis is carefully checked.

Suture. The placement of the sutures is very important to avoid distortion. It is easier to locate the point for the first stitch if the patient is asked to smile or grimace. If the ellipse has been well designed it will lie naturally in a crease and one will see clearly how to close the wound (Fig. 3.4).

Closure is begun with a *deep layer*; a central suture is placed, followed by a suture at each end of the ellipse. This is completed by a sufficient number of sutures to bring the dermis into contact. When the skin is thick and under a certain amount of tension, 4-0 catgut is used for this layer. A 6-0 suture is appropriate when the skin is thin and there is little tension. These dermal-fat sutures are interrupted and inverted, with the knots placed deep (Fig. 3.5).

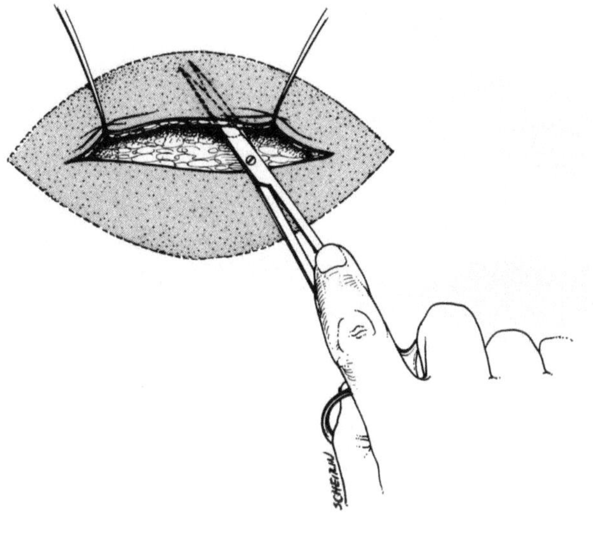

Fig. 3.3. Subcutaneous undermining should be very wide to allow the skin to advance

We prefer not to use nonabsorbable or slow-absorbing sutures when operating on BCCs, since these may give rise to small nodules in the scar in the postoperative period. Catgut is quickly resorbed, and this avoids the risk of confusing a suture reaction with a recurrence.

In the superficial plane we usually use a simple running suture of 6-0 Prolene (Ethicon) (polypropylene monofilament). Running sutures are preferable to interrupted, not only because they are faster but also because they distribute the tension more evenly. They also avoid the placement of numerous knots that can irritate the skin. Certainly, one may elect to use interrupted stitches, or to place several of them and then complete the closure with a running suture (Fig. 3.6). In any case, care must be taken to place the sutures at a consistent depth to ensure precise apposition of the wound edges (Fig. 3.7). Faulty apposition is especially likely to result from a beveled

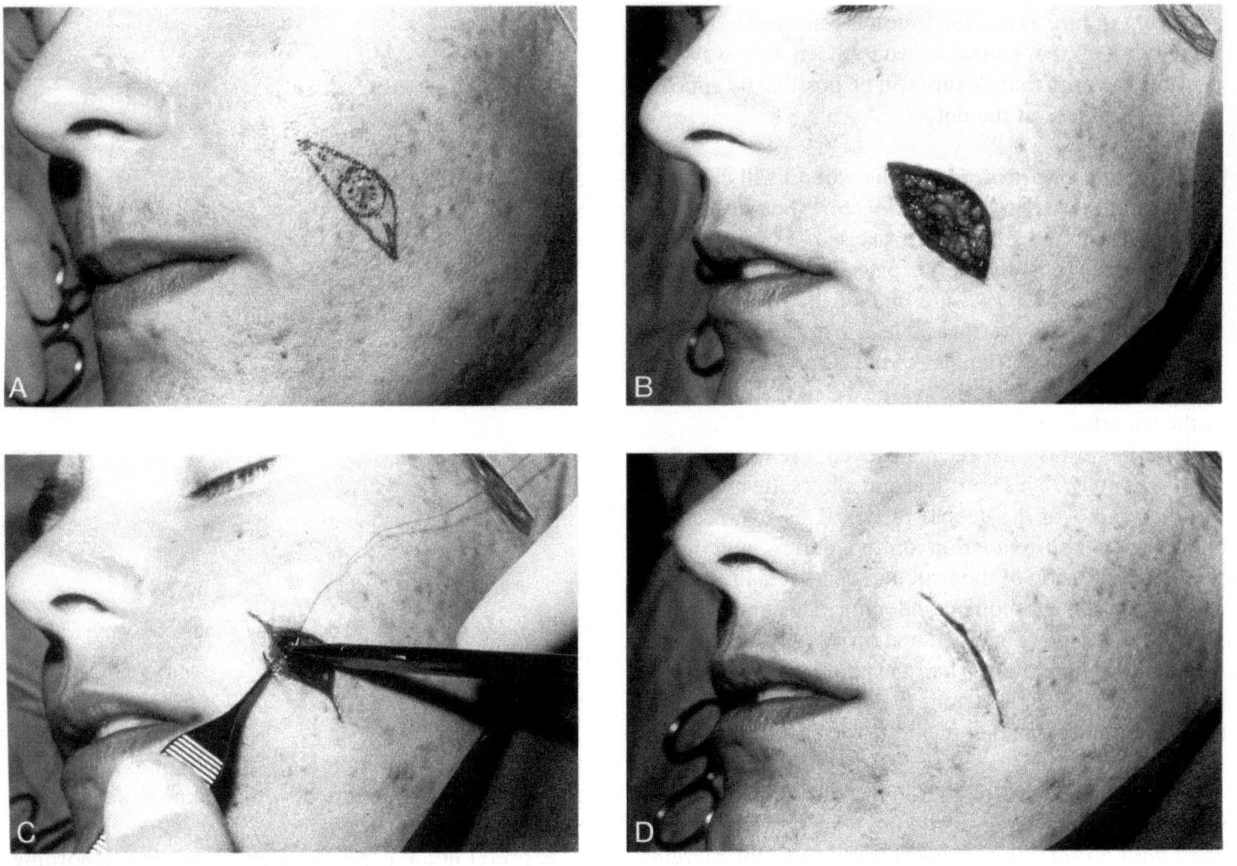

Fig. 3.4 A–H. Elliptical excision in a 28-year-old woman. **A** The ellipse is drawn parallel to natural expression lines which are identified when the patient smiles. **B** After excision and undermining the defect appears large. **C** Placement of inverted sutures of 4-0 catgut. **D** Closure of the dermis-fat plane should bring the margins into contact. **E** A simple running suture of 6-0 polypropylene. **F** The suture should approximate the edges precisely without being too tight. **G** The result at 10 months. **H** Two years post-op

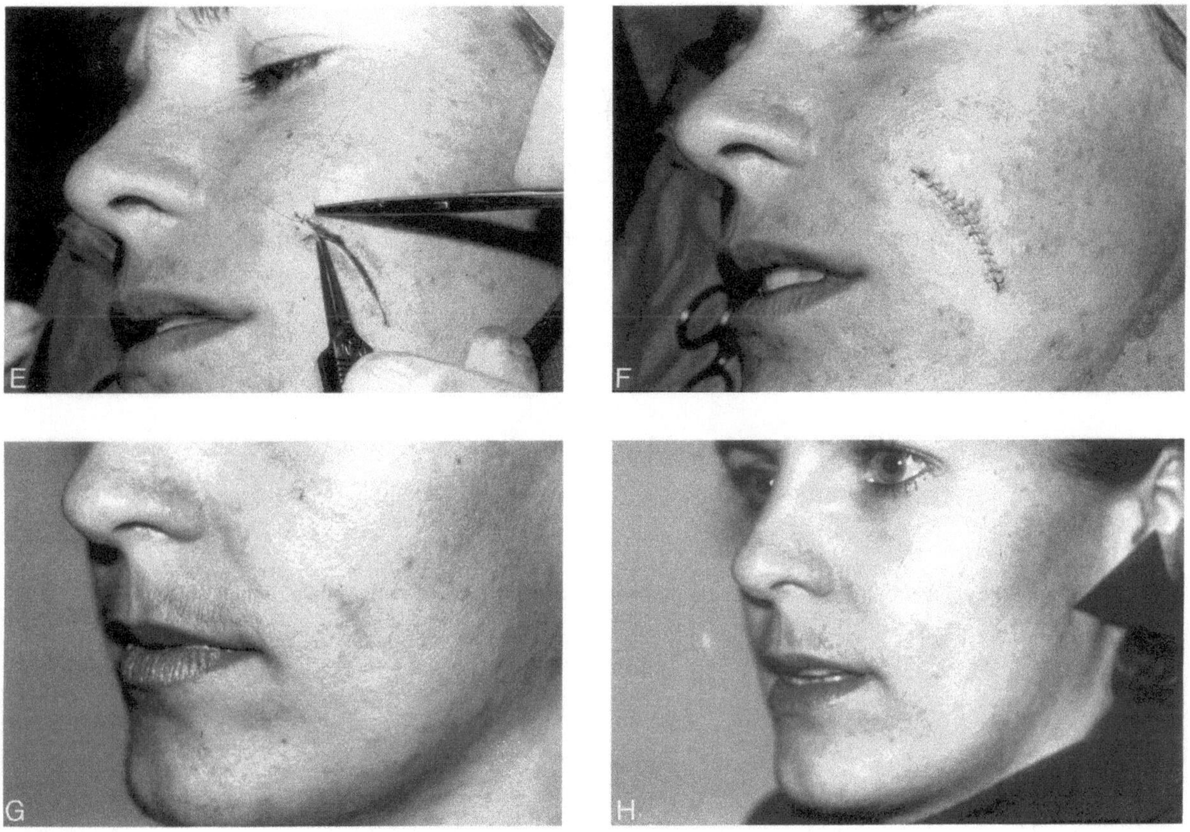
E
F
G
H

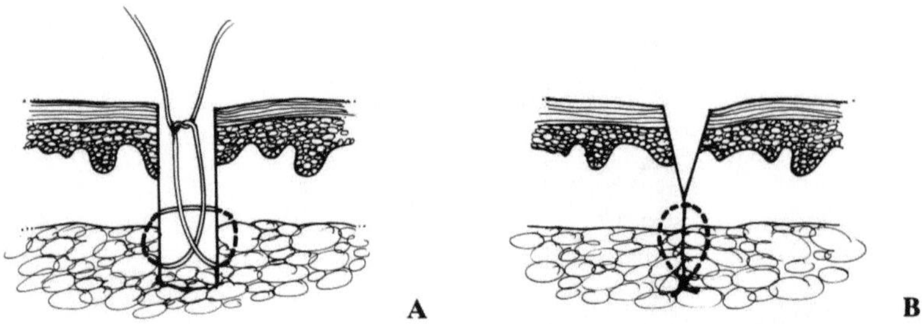

Fig. 3.5 A, B. Closure of the deep layer. **A** The inverted suture approximates the deep dermis and fat (when it is present). **B** The knot is deep

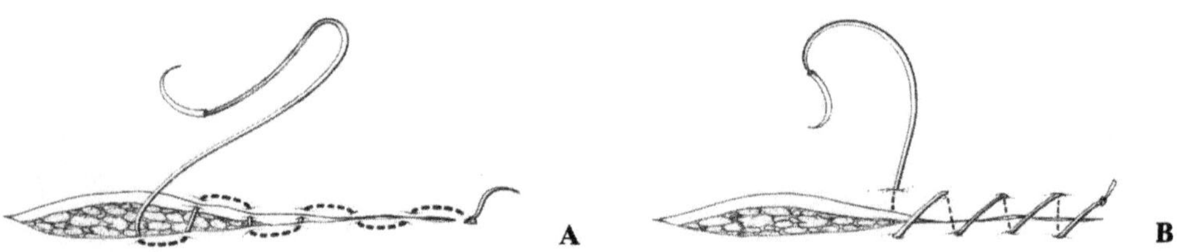

Fig. 3.6. The superficial layer can be closed with a running subcuticular suture (**A**) or a simple running suture (**B**)

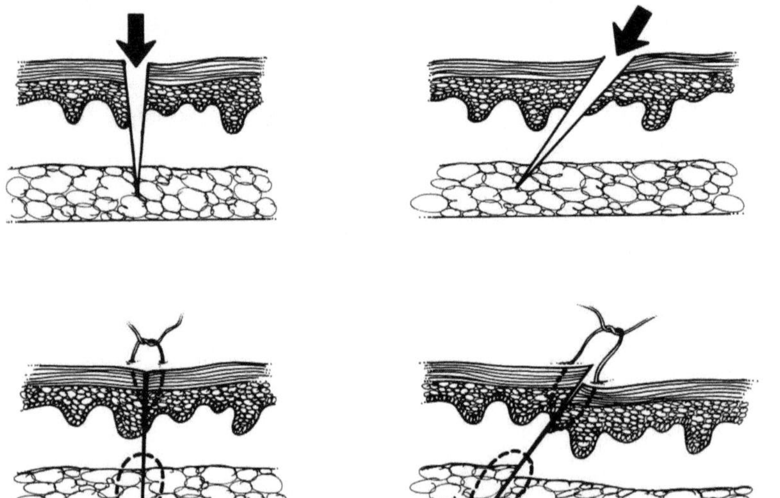

Fig. 3.7 A, B. Precise apposition of the wound margins is indispensable. **A** A perpendicular incision permits perfect apposition. **B** A beveled incision allows one margin to slide over the other, leading to a step deformity

incision, and may not be obvious when the skin is closed with a simple running suture.

When there is a significant degree of tension on the wound, as with a large elliptical excision in the cheek, it is advisable to use a running subcuticular suture of 5-0 Prolene followed by several interrupted sutures of 6-0 Prolene (Fig. 3.6).

The 6-0 sutures are removed after several days and replaced with Steristrips (3M Laboratories), while the subcuticular suture may be left in place for 3 weeks. This will decrease the spreading of the scar.

Dressing. When the wound has been closed with a running subcuticular suture we place Steristrips transversely across the incision and secure the ends of the suture with several strips as well.

In most cases we apply an antibiotic-hydrocortisone ointment to the wound and follow this with a pressure dressing. The latter is useful in preventing hematoma when a large area has been undercut. A sufficiently thick layer of folded gauze sponges is placed over the area of the dissection and is held under tension with 3-cm Elastoplast (Fisch Laboratories), after the skin has been cleaned with ether.

Postoperative Care. The patient is instructed to remove the pressure dressing later that evening or the following morning. An analgesic such as Doliprane (Bottu Laboratories) is prescribed and the patient is warned against taking aspirin or aspirin-containing products.

The wound is cleaned twice daily with hydrogen peroxide and a cotton-tipped applicator. The patient removes all crusts and fibrin deposits and then applies a thin layer of an antibiotic-hydrocortisone ointment such as Cidermex (Specia Laboratories).

The sutures are removed as early as possible to prevent the development of suture marks. These will appear on about the 6th day, especially when there is tension on the wound and interrupted sutures have been used. It is advisable to use Steristrips for several days after the sutures have been removed.

Wound Healing. The scar is often fine and smooth at the time of suture removal, but frequently it will become thick, red, and pruritic after 2 or 3 weeks. The patient must be warned that this is a normal development (Fig. 3.8).

Apart from minimizing exposure to the sun, the patient should massage the scar with hydrocortisone cream if pruritis develops. This must remain a short-term treatment, as we have seen skin atrophy and telangiectasias after a number of weeks of such therapy.

The inflammation will begin to recede at the end of the 2nd month. Nevertheless, the final result of a flat, supple scar is not usually attained until 6–12 months following surgery. Occasionally, this process takes longer and may produce a keloid scar, but this usually resolves spontaneously without it being necessary to resort to steroid injections.

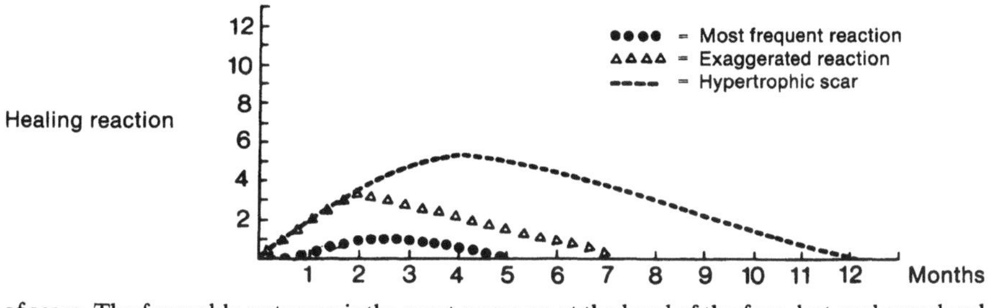

Fig. 3.8. Different types of evolution of scars. The favorable outcome is the most common at the level of the face, but prolonged and excessive hypertrophic reactions are possible

Correct Orientation of the Elliptical Excision (Fig. 3.1)

The cheek: local skin laxity makes this a favorable area, and the ellipse is easily drawn in the smile lines. It must be made long enough to avoid the creation of dog-ears (see Fig. 4.1, p. 27).

The temporal area: this is also favorable, since the excision is placed in the radiating wrinkles of the crow's feet. One must avoid the frontal branch of the facial nerve located between the end of the eyebrow and the temporal hairs, under the muscle layer (see Fig. 4.42, p. 76).

The eyelids: this is a good area for closure of limited defects in patients with excess skin. The natural folds of the lids serve as a guide for the excision (see Fig. 4.27, p. 61). For low-lying lesions one should try to place the scar at the junction of the fine skin of the lid and the thicker cheek skin. The skin is undermined above the m. orbicularis.

The forehead: at first glance, the forehead would appear to be favored by its wrinkles (see Fig. 4.36, p. 70). However, even in the setting of skin laxity, a unilateral excision may produce permanent elevation of the eyebrow. It may also displace the horizontal frontal wrinkles, and this is very visible when the eyebrows are raised. Even moderate skin defects of the forehead are best repaired by an H-flap, which will be discussed later (see Fig. 4.37, p. 71).

The nose: only rarely can an elliptical excision be made in the nose, because there is very little laxity and distortions are readily produced.

The lips: elliptical excisions can occasionally be oriented radially around the mouth, but most often a portion of red lip will have to be excised to avoid creating a deformity (see Fig. 4.8, p. 37).

In conclusion, the elliptical excision gives good results when (a) the ellipse is sufficiently long and properly oriented (Fig. 3.1), (b) adequate undermining permits true advancement rather than a simple approximation of the edges, and (c) careful suturing with correct placement of the stitches produces perfect epithelial contact.

This "minor surgery" requires considerable precision and appropriate materials in order to be executed well. A closure that would be satisfactory on the back is unacceptable in the face, where the best possible result must be obtained for the patient.

These procedures are always carried out in an operating room with the help of an assistant who places the skin under tension, retracts, and cuts the sutures. Of course, one can do without an assistant. In the 1960s an elderly country surgeon told me that his predecessor had been accustomed to performing gastrectomies alone with the help of self-retaining retractors and traction sutures. One can do the same with elliptical skin excisions, but in this case the use of fine self-retaining retractors is strongly recommended, particularly to obtain hemostasis after wide undercutting.

Repairs Using Plastic Surgery Techniques, Grafts and Flaps

When primary closure would result in excessive tension or produce a deformity, more complex techniques of repair must be considered.

Split-thickness Skin Graft. These grafts are harvested with a skin-grafting knife or a dermatome and may vary in thickness (Fig. 3.9). They have no place in the repair of small defects of the face because their color and texture are too different from those of the cervicofacial skin. The split-thickness graft maintains the pigmentation of the donor site, and the cervicofacial region has a different color than the rest of the body due to its rich vascularity. The texture of the split-thickness graft is different due to the absence of pilosebaceous skin adnexa. The graft is smooth and occasionally shiny, and it is therefore difficult to hide.

It is only in exceptional cases, such as with a large superficial BCC in an elderly patient, that such a graft could be used, and then only in the interest of simplicity. Even here, the graft could be harvested from the scalp after shaving and infiltration with saline. The color match is superior, although often the orifices of the hair follicles are visible.

Although it is technically possible we are not in favor of harvesting split-thickness grafts from the neck for two reasons: (a) it may produce a visible scar or even

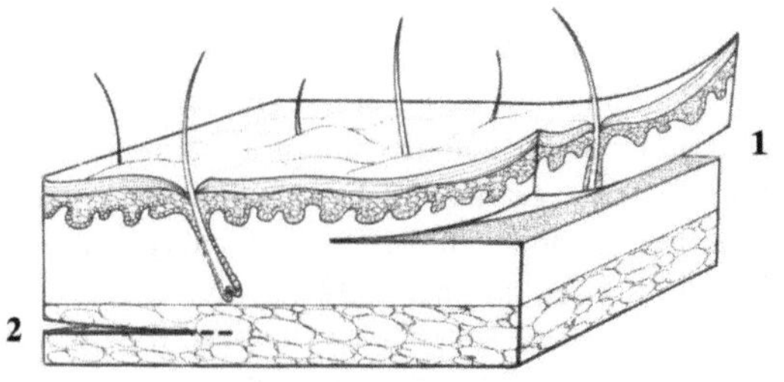

Fig. 3.9. Skin grafts are (*1*) split thickness when they contain only part of the dermis. The donor site will re-epithelialize spontaneously, but the graft contains no skin adnexae; (*2*) full thickness when the entire dermis is harvested with the graft. The donor site will not re-epithelialize and must be closed

contracture if healing is not perfect, and (b) it is easy to harvest a full-thickness graft in this area. The medial aspect of the arm may also be used for this purpose if necessary.

Full-thickness Skin Graft. These are preferably harvested in the retroauricular area where the scar is not visible (Fig. 3.9). Large grafts may be taken from the supraclavicular region, but at the cost of a visible scar. Grafts can sometimes be obtained by a vertical preauricular excision. Skin can be taken from the upper eyelid to repair the contralateral lid.

Although the full-thickness skin graft appears to be a simple method it is in fact difficult and the results are unpredictable. Despite meticulous technique it can be complicated by partial or complete necrosis. Even several drops of blood beneath the graft will prevent revascularization. The long-term result is unpredictable because, although some are nearly invisible, many grafts remain extremely conspicuous.

Execution of the full-thickness graft requires very careful technique. The recipient site must be smooth and well vascularized, and hemostasis must be perfect. The donor site must be chosen with care; its color and texture should resemble as closely as possible that of the area of the defect. For example, retroauricular skin is very different from the skin of the mastoid region.

In certain areas it is advisable to enlarge the defect to have it correspond to an anatomic unit; e.g., a graft of the upper lip may optimally be extended to the nasolabial fold.

The graft should be applied under slight tension and the edges perfectly approximated to the surrounding skin. We use simple sutures of 5-0 Prolene followed by a running suture of 6-0 Prolene. Contact between the graft and the recipient bed is essential, and mattress sutures may be required when the contour of the recipient site is irregular. This carries the risk of injuring a vessel and causing bleeding beneath the graft.

Since 1982 we have frequently used a biologic glue (Tissucol, Immuno France) composed of human fibrinogen and bovine thrombin. This adhesive produces immediate graft–bed adherence and considerably increases the chances for a successful take. The glue is completely resorbed and does not inhibit vascularization, provided that it has been applied as a thin layer.

A tie-over dressing is indispensable; it is fixed in place with the long end of the interrupted Prolene sutures. Further security is provided by a pressure dressing to avoid any displacement. It is important to immobilize the grafted zone during the early postoperative period, and we do not hesitate to institute temporary intermaxillary fixation with a steel wire for grafts near the mouth and the lower cheek. The dressing is removed on the 5th day and a uniform pink color indicates a satisfactory take. Dark areas indicate small hematomas which may cause localized slough of the graft. Significant hematoma is evacuated, but very small collections are best left alone, as attempted drainage will not be helpful.

It should be evident that the procedure is a delicate one if the best chances for success are to be assured, and that the immediate and long-term results are often unpredictable. Therefore, in our opinion, the full-thickness graft should be planned only when no satisfactory local flap is available.

Composite Grafts. These are grafts that contain several tissue elements and, in the present context, consist of skin and cartilage. These composite grafts are harvested from the ear for reconstruction of the ala of the nose (Fig. 3.10). Harvest of a wedge-shaped graft leaves a defect which, when carefully repaired, leaves virtually no deformity. It yields a graft which sandwiches a plate of

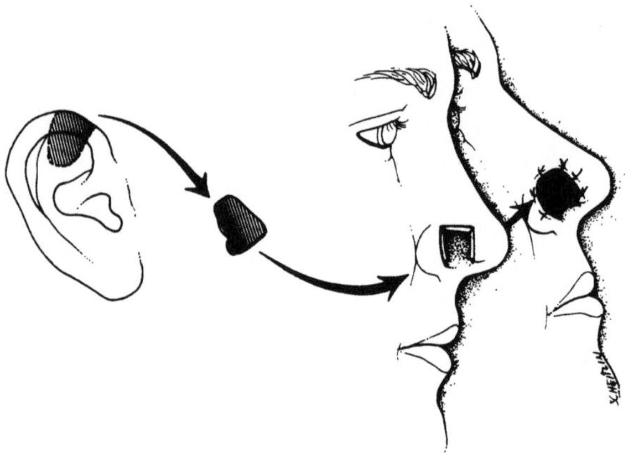

Fig. 3.10. The composite graft. A full-thickness nostril defect may be reconstructed with an auricular graft consisting of a layer of cartilage sandwiched between two layers of skin

cartilage between two layers of skin, and which is perfect for reconstruction of the alar margin. Our teacher Claude Dufourmentel was particularly adept at achieving complete take of large grafts. We have had several partial failures, although they healed in time and may be revised later (see Fig. 4.26, p. 58). Perhaps we did not pay sufficient attention to the Russian author who recommended having the patient swallow a large glass of vodka to produce vasodilatation.

A composite eyelid graft harvested from a normal lid is very useful in the reconstruction of the lid margin.

Local Flaps. It should be emphasized at the outset that these represent the ideal solution for the majority of repairs following excision of BCCs of the face. There are many useful local flaps, and the choice depends on several factors:

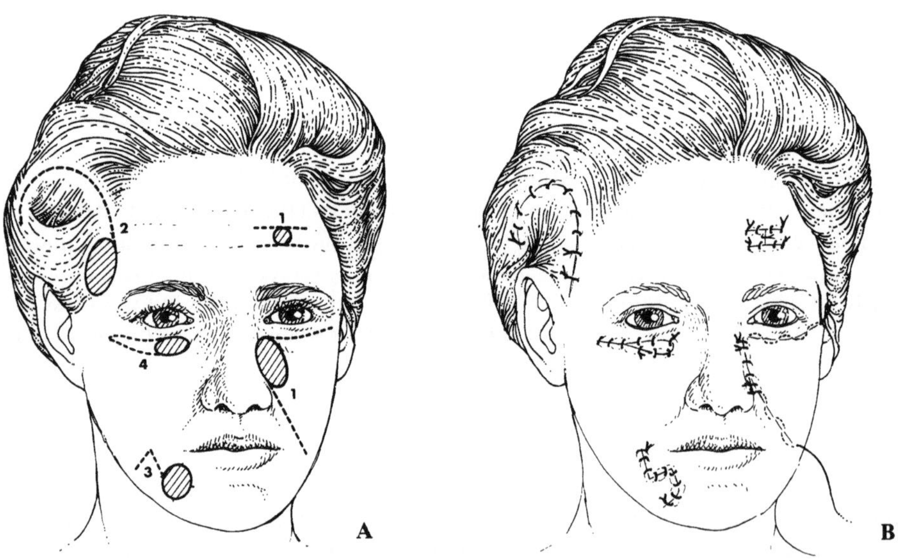

Fig. 3.11 A, B. Different local flaps that can be used in the face: **A** excision; **B** closure. *1*, Double advancement flaps; *2*, rotation flap; *3*, Dufourmentel LLL-flap; *4*, Dufourmentel kite flap

1. The location of skin laxity relative to the defect
2. The direction of the skin lines and the shape of the defect
3. The texture of the missing skin and that of the various possible flaps

Following is a review of alternative local flaps that can be used in the face.

For the *advancement flap*, following wide undermining, two incisions are made perpendicular to the axis of the defect to allow advancement of two rectangular flaps (Fig. 3.11). The incisions are closed by compensating the unequal lengths of the wound edges, or by resecting Burow's triangles from the external margin.

This flap is indicated when the incisions can be placed in wrinkle lines or along natural anatomic borders, as in the medial part of the cheek. The H-flap is a double advancement flap that is especially effective for repairs in the forehead (Color Plate IA and D, p. 108).

After wide undercutting, a *rotation (Imre) flap* provides the necessary tissue to fill the defect. The scar is long relative to the defect and this technique is indicated at the junction of scalp and skin where the scar can be hidden in the hair (Fig. 3.12 and Fig. 4.43, p. 77).

The Dufourmentel LLL-flap is a *transposition flap* where an adjacent triangle of excess skin is transposed across an intervening zone of normal skin. The LLL-flap is very versatile and allows an even distribution of tension. It creates a dog-ear and the flap must be planned so that its excision lies in a skin fold (Fig. 3.13). It is useful for small repairs of such as areas the nose, as well as for large reconstructions, e.g., of the cheek (Fig. 4.14, p. 44 and Color Plate IID, p. 109).

The kite flap on a subcutaneous pedicle (Dufourmentel) is the latest generation of local flaps, allowing the advancement of adjacent tissue with minimal scars and deformity (Dufourmentel and Talaat 1971; Herbert and Degens 1975). All the preceding flaps are vascularized by a skin pedicle and involve subcutaneous undermining. The kite flap is radically different in that the skin is cut completely around the flap, and the blood is supplied via the subcutaneous tissue. Therefore, undermining is limited, gradual, and careful, preserving central or lateral subcutaneous pedicles. The skin island must advance into the

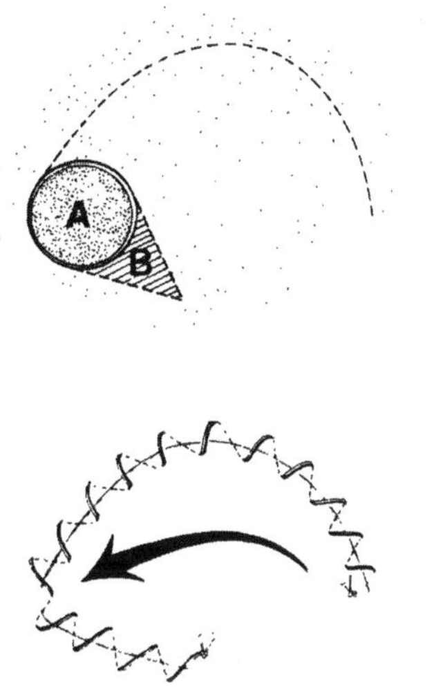

Fig. 3.12. Rotation flap. Triangle *B* is excised. The dotted area is undermined to allow insetting of the flap and suture of the unequal margins

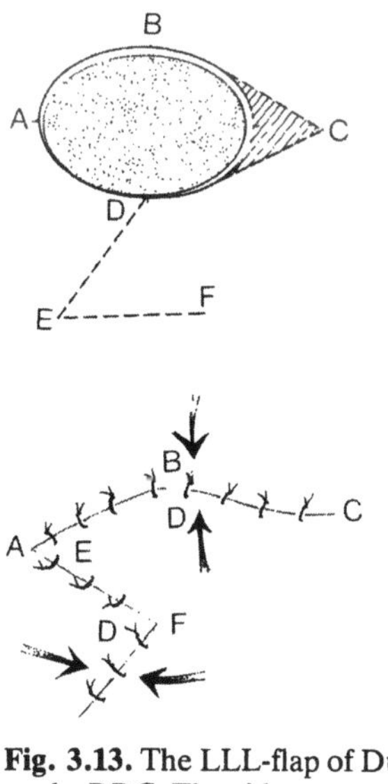

Fig. 3.13. The LLL-flap of Dufourmentel. Line *DE* bisects the angle *BDC*. The sides are equal in length to *AB* and *AD*. The flap is transposed over the area *ADE* to fill the defect. A triangle is excised to point *C*. The flap has the advantage of distributing tension particularly well

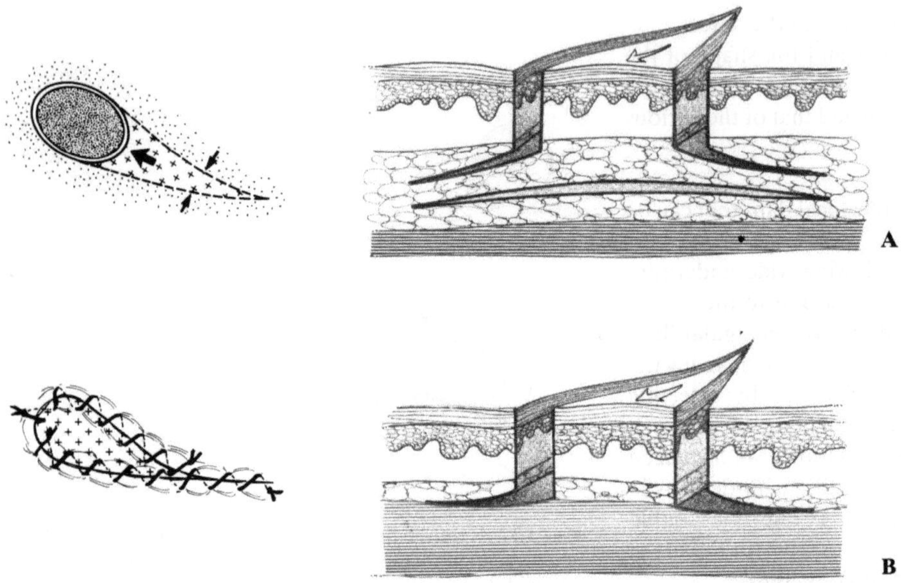

Fig. 3.14 A, B. The kite flap of Dufourmentel. Adjacent skin, roughly corresponding to half an ellipse, is advanced on a subcutaneous pedicle. The skin may be based on subcutaneous tissue (**A**), in which case the pedicle is located laterally, or on musculocutaneous perforators (**B**). The muscle advances easily with the skin

defect without tension. Peripheral undercutting will facilitate closure of the donor site (Fig. 3.14), which must be carefully chosen with reference to local skin laxity and the direction of the skin folds.

The flap can be small or very large and provides excellent aesthetic results (Fig. 4.28, p. 61), especially in the eyelids and around the nasolabial fold. This is due to the fact that the flap advances directly without rotation or distortion. The difficulty is that the flap must be freed sufficiently from the subcutaneous tissues to permit tensionless advancement and must at the same time maintain the blood supply.

In addition to these flaps which are widely useful, there are two others which are of regional importance: the frontonasal flap for the nose (Fig. 4.15, p. 45) (Marchac 1970; Marchac and Alkhateb 1974); the cheek-advancement flap for reconstruction of the lower eyelid (Mustardé 1966).

Distant Flaps. These are rarely employed in the surgery of BCCs, but in certain cases they may be indicated.

Pedicled on the rich supraorbital vasculature, the forehead flap provides forehead skin for coverage of the middle third of the face. Its range is primarily determined by the height of the forehead, and we prefer an obliquely oriented flap to lengthen the reach. Usually, the pedicle is returned to the donor site secondarily. In certain cases the skin can be transferred as an island on a subcutaneous pedicle which is tunneled or on which the adjacent skin is adjusted (Fig. 4.19, p. 51).

The Washio retroauricular temporal flap (Washio 1969; Maillard and Montandon 1982) allows the transfer to the

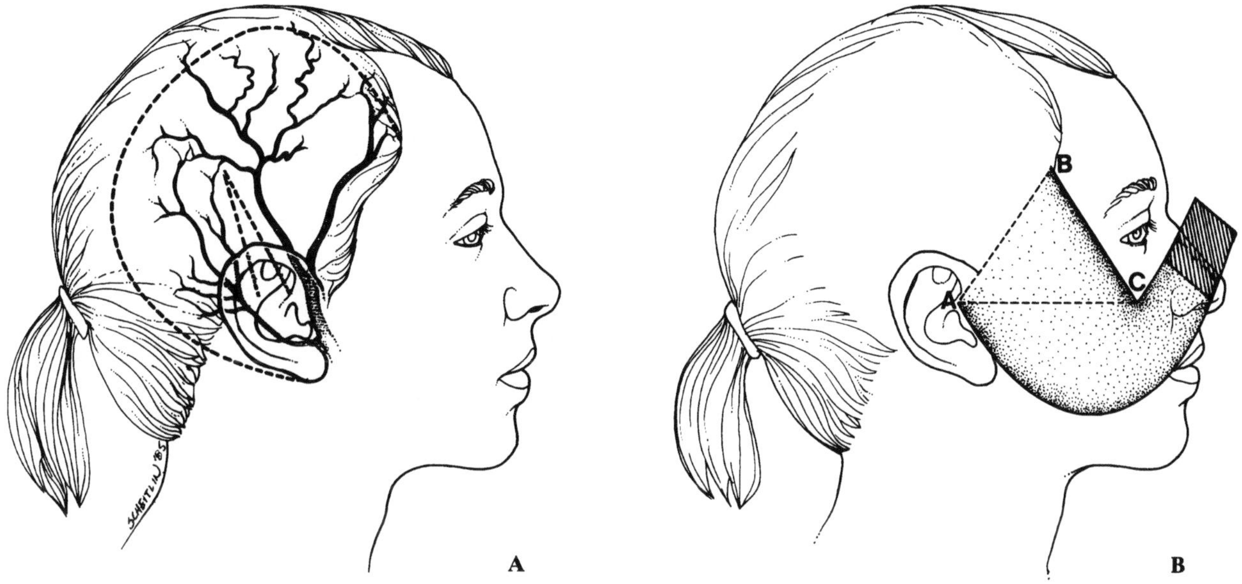

Fig. 3.15 A, B. The Washio flap (**A**). This flap permits the transfer to the face of retroauricular and mastoid skin on a temporal pedicle which is returned to the donor site secondarily. The absence of visible scars is a great advantage of this relatively complex procedure with its double folding of the pedicle (**B**)

face of all the retroauricular and mastoid skin, based on a wide temporal pedicle which is folded twice. The flap is very bulky, but when returned to the donor site after 15–20 days the scars are hidden in the scalp (Fig. 3.15). The flap is based on anastomoses between the temporal and posterior auricular arteries.

In *myocutaneous flaps* the blood supply to the skin is derived from musculocutaneous perforating vessels. The most relevant is the platysma flap which allows transfer of supraclavicular skin to the face. This is an one-stage procedure, and the donor site is closed primarily after wide undermining (Tessier 1974). In certain large resections one can use the deltopectoral flap.

Following extremely extensive resections, *free flaps* with microanastomoses to the facial or temporal arteries may be required.

The recently developed technique of *skin expansion* (Radovan 1984) must be mentioned here. A silicone expander is placed beneath adjacent normal skin and progressively inflated with saline through a one-way valve. This skin is expanded over a period of 4–6 weeks and can be used as a flap or full-thickness skin graft (Fig. 4.21, p. 54). This technique is not indicated for the great majority of BCCs because of the delay it imposes and because classical techniques can usually provide immediate repair. Nevertheless, skin expansion has a role in certain difficult cases: (a) following an extensive resection where a split-thickness skin graft is used to provide temporary coverage; (b) in cases where surgery is not judged to be urgent, such as with slowly growing tumors or areas of radiodermatitis which are at risk for malignant degeneration.

Chapter 4 Repair by Region

Here we will review the various anatomic regions of the face and the techniques of repair that are particularly appropriate to each area.

The Cheek

This is a relatively large homogeneous area characterized by significant laxity beginning at about 30 years of age. It is not an anatomically dangerous region, since backward the parotid gland, anteriorely the facial nerve branches and parotid duct are protected usually by a good thickness of subcutaneous tissue. Operative planning must take into account the expression lines that run parallel to the nasolabial fold. Contour irregularities such as dog-ears are very visible on this slightly convex surface. The skin often has dilated pores which compromise the quality of the scar.

Elliptical excisions are ideally suited to the cheek area because of local skin laxity and the wrinkles that can be used to hide the scar (Figs. 4.1, 3.1, and 3.4). Excessive tension must be avoided as it can result in widening of the scar and in asymmetry due to softening the ipsilateral nasolabial fold.

Flap repair is usually indicated when the defect exceeds approximately 7 mm in the young patient and 15 mm in the adult. The kite flap is the one most frequently used (Figs. 4.2 and 4.3), while the LLL-flap is indicated occasionally. Large resections may necessitate the use of classical cervical rotation flaps (Fig. 6.1, p. 98) or the platysma myocutaneous flap.

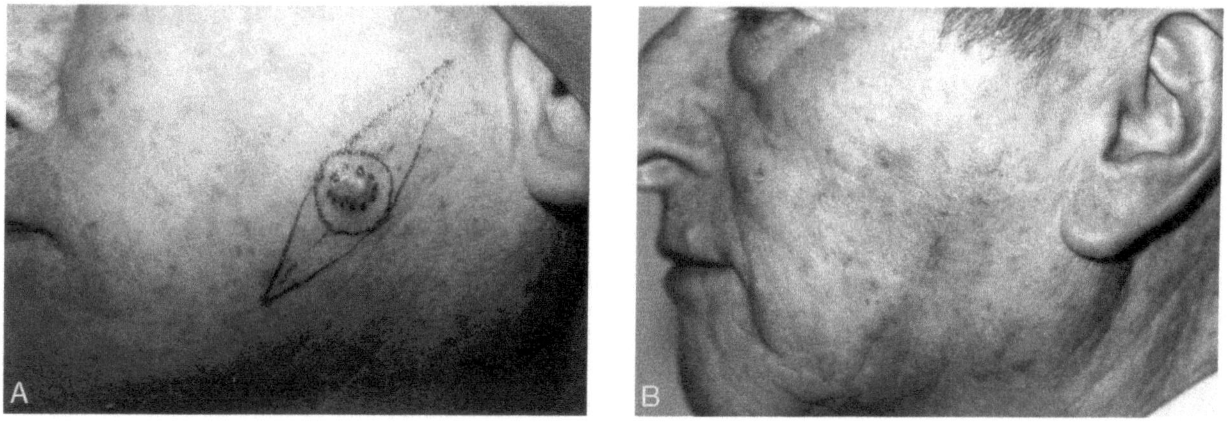

Fig. 4.1. A Elliptical excision of a BCC of the cheek in a 76-year-old man. Note the orientation of the skin wrinkles. **B** Appearance at 2 months

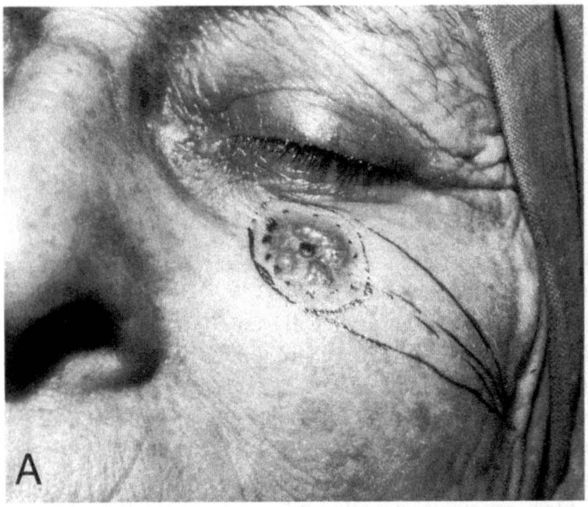

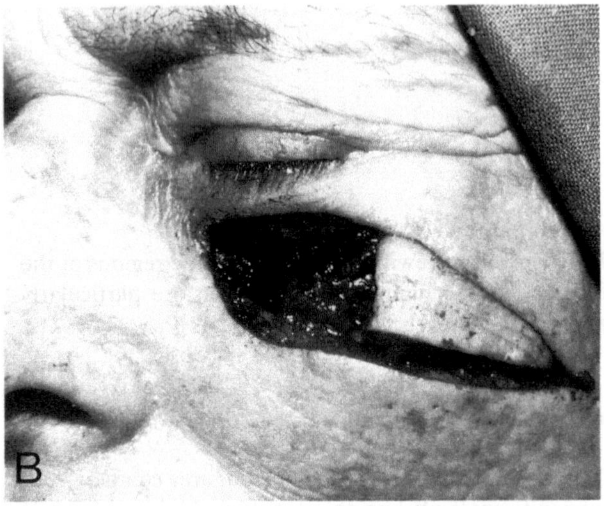

Fig. 4.2 A–E. The kite flap. **A** A 70-year-old patient with a BCC of the cheek close to the lower eyelid of 2 years duration, untreated. **B** and **C** The kite flap is mobilized on a pedicle of subcutaneous fat. **D** The definitive histologic sections revealed inadequate margins medially, and at 7 days re-excision was carried out and the flap simply readvanced. **E** Five years later there has been no recurrence and the aesthetic result is considered "good"

The full-thickness skin graft may be indicated to resurface widespread lesions. Figure 4.4 shows such a graft in a patient who had received radiotherapy for a hemangioma and developed radiodermatitis and multiple BCCs. All the cheek skin was removed, ruling out the use of local flaps. One option would have been a free dorsalis pedis flap which transfers thin skin of sometimes acceptable color. We preferred a large full-thickness skin graft which provides an equivalent or superior result with far less complex surgery. The ideal donor site is the neck, but for very large grafts the medial aspect of the arm is the best alternative because (a) its color is not very different from that of the face, and (b) the donor site is either closed primarily or grafted and is generally hidden.

The junction between ala and cheek has a poor reputation because of high rates of recurrence. This has not been confirmed in the present series (see p. 86), perhaps because of the wide excisions carried out in this area. The skin of the fold is thick, and an adequate excision must be both wide and deep. However, the laxity of the cheek

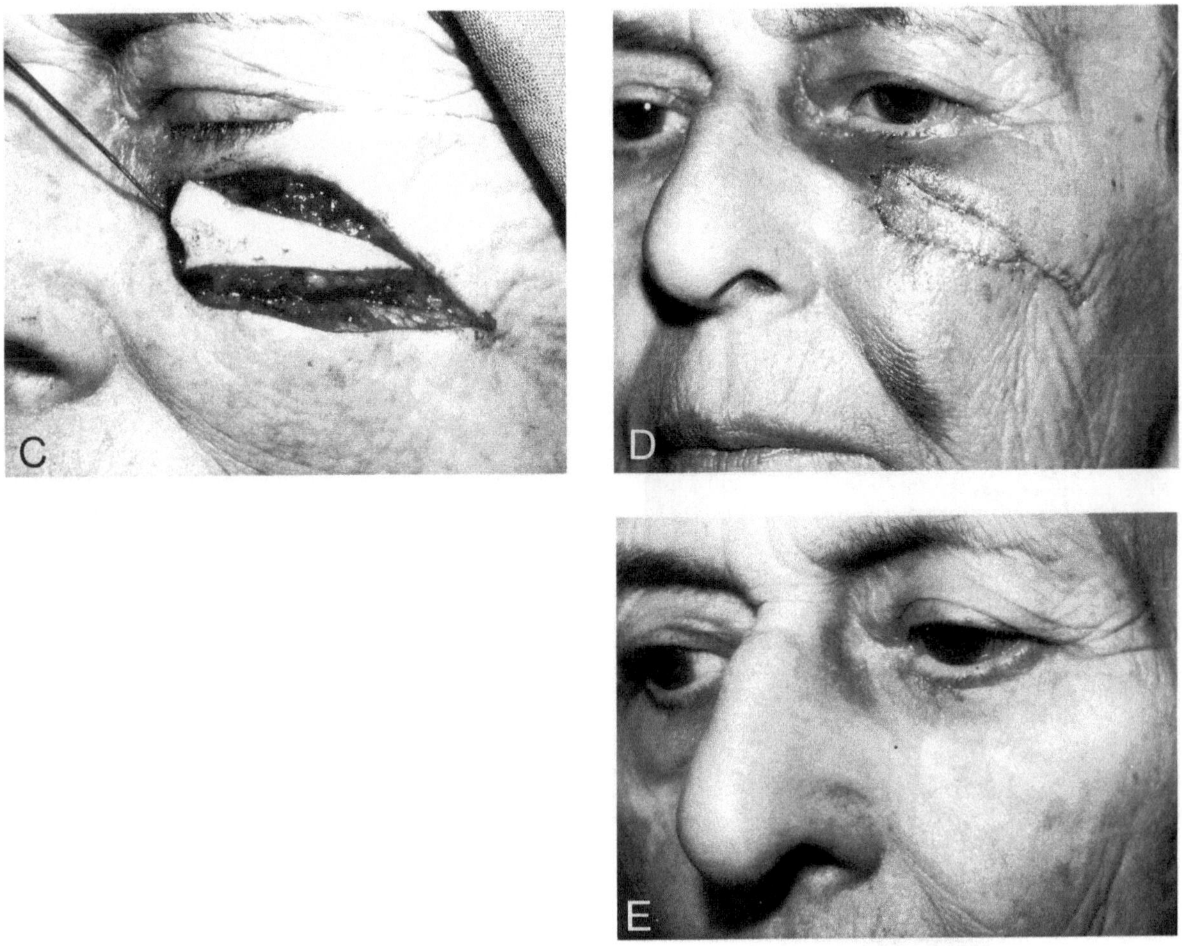

skin facilitates repair, which can be carried out with an advancement flap or an LLL-flap (Fig. 4.5).

The nasolabial fold represents the border between the nose and the cheek and lower eyelid. The angular artery, a branch of the facial artery, runs in this area and frequently must be sacrificed in local tumor resections. The looseness of the local skin allows use of advancement flaps (Color Plate 1D, p 108), the LLL-flap (Fig. 4.6), or the kite flap. One must take care not to place excessive tension on the lower eyelid.

In the area of the lower nasolabial fold natural skin laxity must be preserved to avoid creating asymmetry. Therefore, one or even two kite flaps (Fig. 4.7) are particularly indicated.

The preauricular area is distinguished by the presence of the parotid gland. The subcutaneous tissue is sometimes thin and firmly adherent to the underlying gland, so that local flaps pedicled on subcutaneous tissue are best avoided. Elliptical excisions provide excellent results when undermining is extended widely into the cheek (Fig. 3.2).

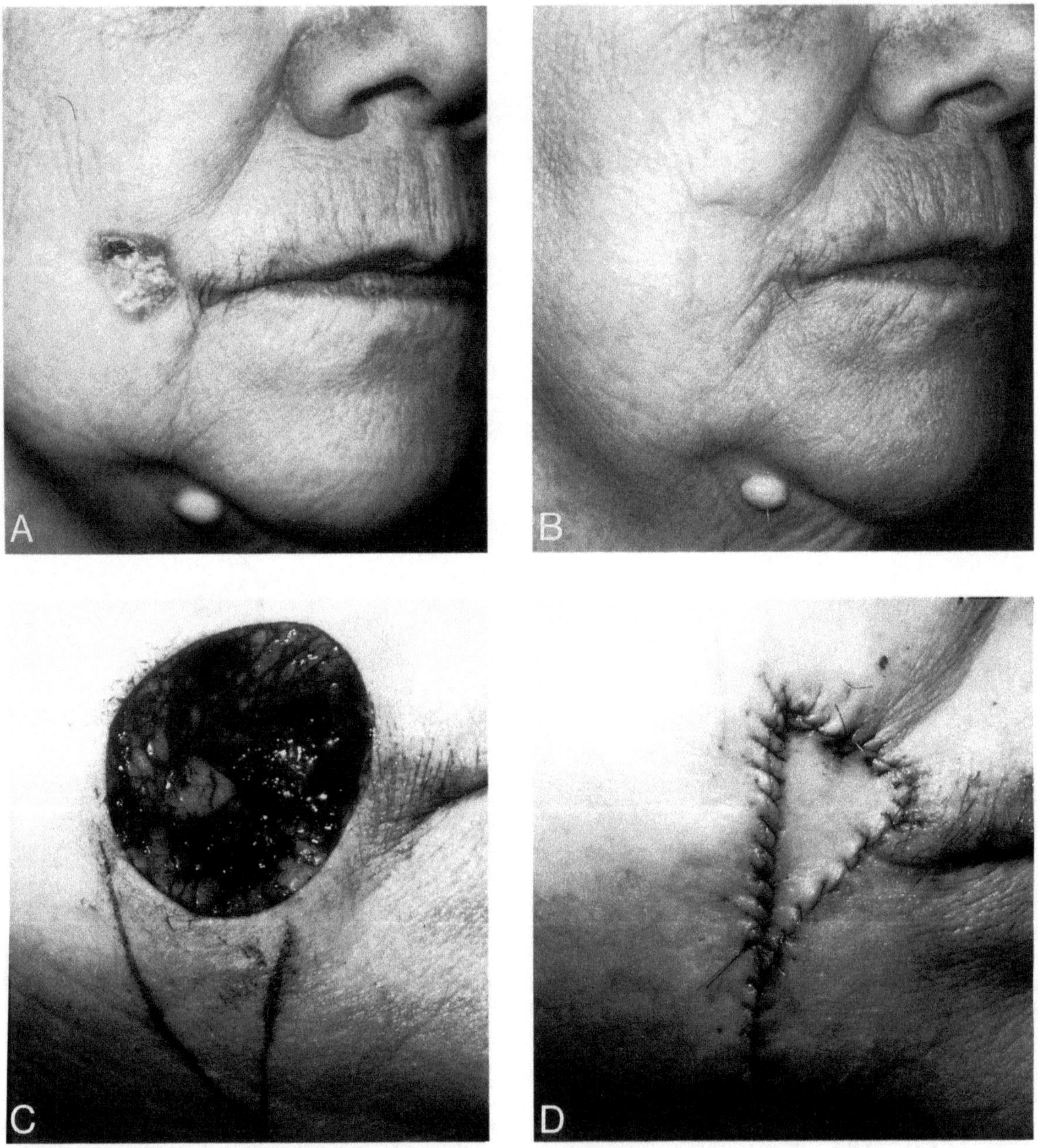

Fig. 4.3 A–D. The kite flap. **A** An 83-year-old patient with an untreated sclerosing BCC. **B** Nine months following repair. **C** and **D** The kite flap is designed below the defect to take advantage of the skin laxity in the lower cheek. This method of closure avoids placing tension on the oral commissure

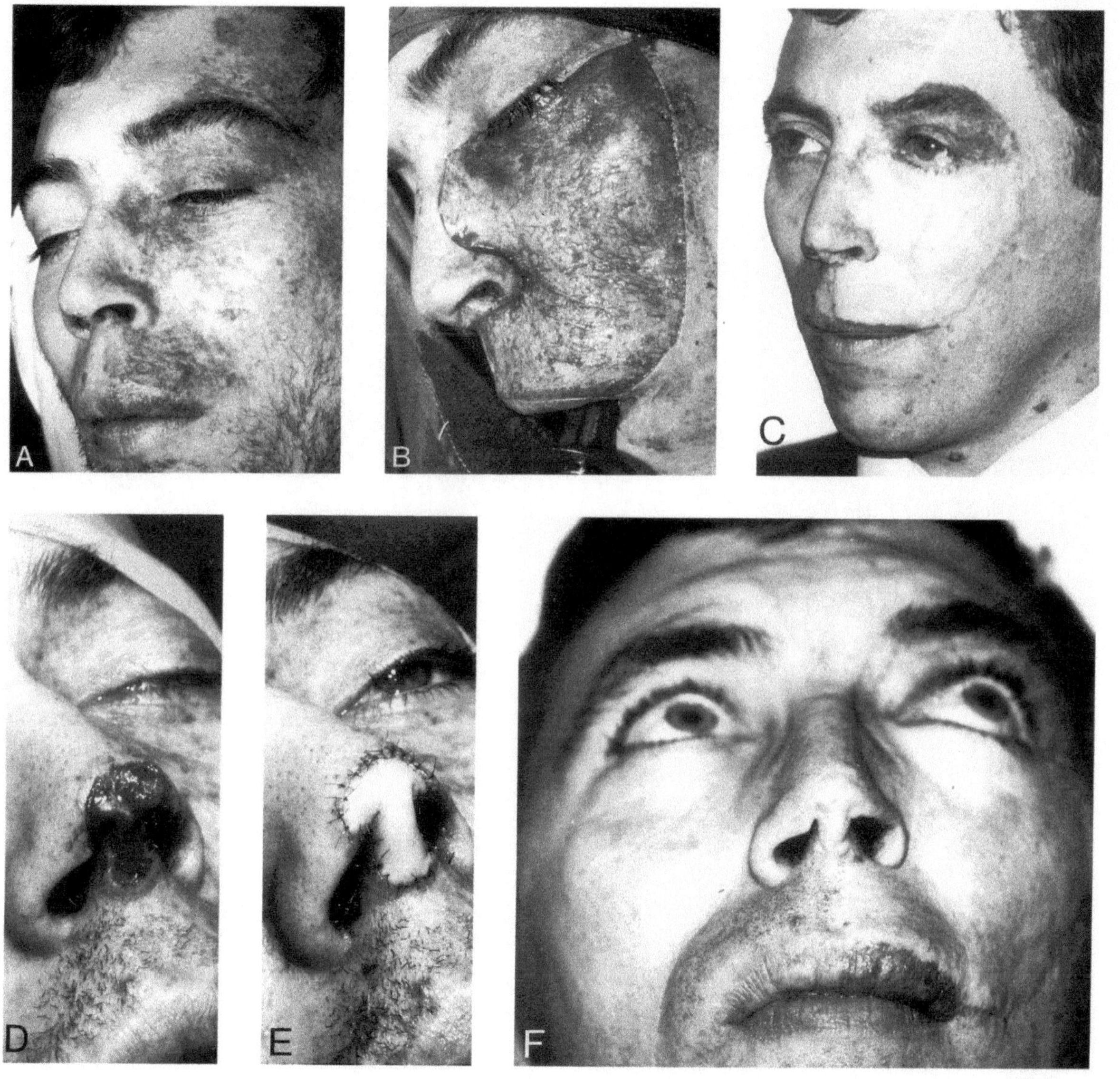

Fig. 4.4 A–F. Full-thickness skin graft. **A** A 25-year-old patient who had undergone therapeutic irradiation of a hemangioma on the left side of the face in childhood. A BCC has developed on the tip of the nose and there is diffuse radiodermatitis of the cheek. **B** The cheek skin has been excised. **C** Three years following coverage with a full-thickness skin graft taken from the medial aspect of the arm. **D** and **E** Excision of the tumor of the nasal tip and repair with a graft from the ear lobule. **F** Appearance at 3 years

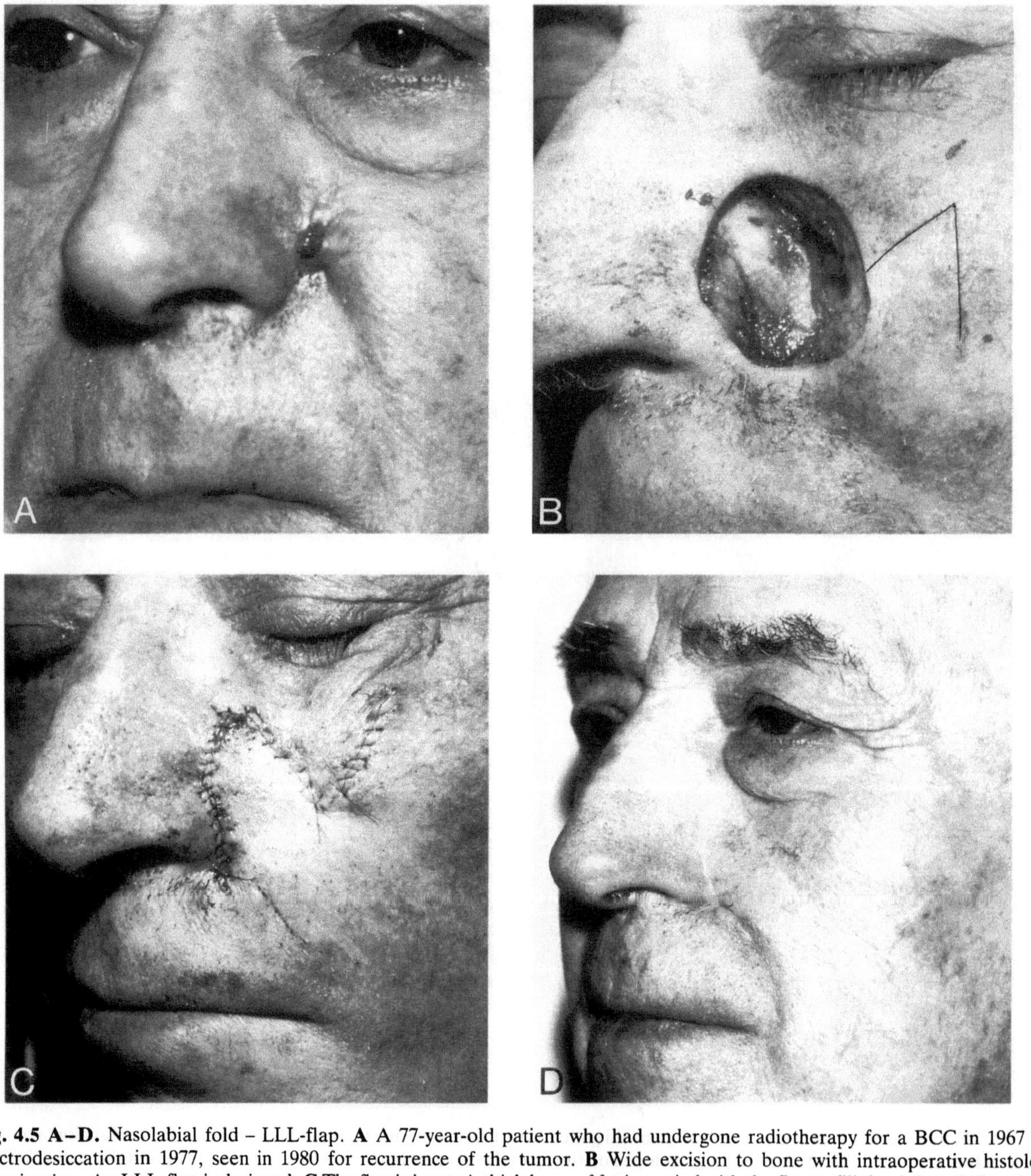

Fig. 4.5 A–D. Nasolabial fold – LLL-flap. **A** A 77-year-old patient who had undergone radiotherapy for a BCC in 1967 and electrodesiccation in 1977, seen in 1980 for recurrence of the tumor. **B** Wide excision to bone with intraoperative histologic examination. An LLL-flap is designed. **C** The flap is inset. A thick layer of fat is carried with the flap to fill the defect. **D** Result at 3 years. There has been no recurrence of the tumor, and the aesthetic result is judged "good"

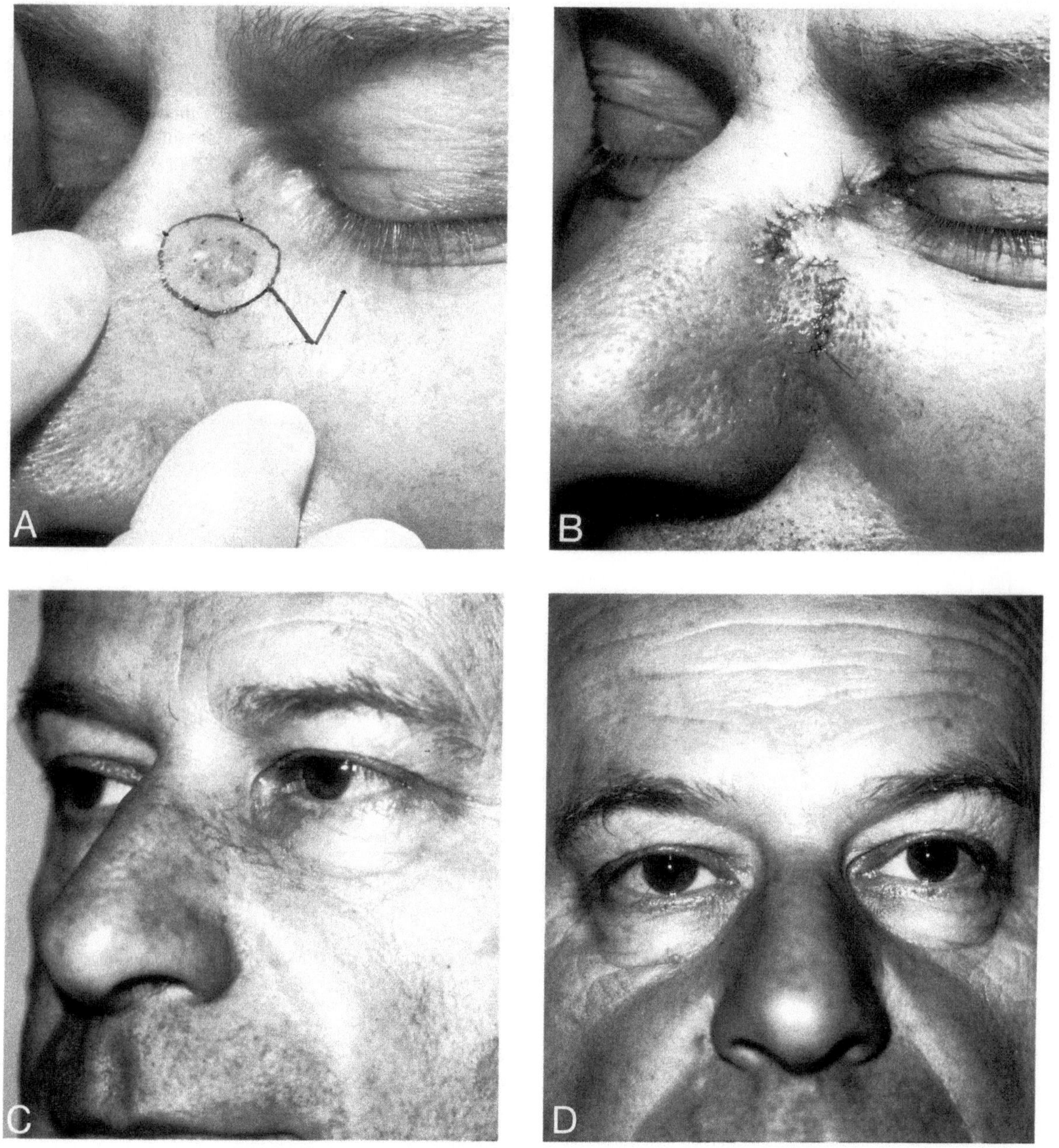

Fig. 4.6 A–D. Nasolabial fold – LLL-flap. **A** A 58-year-old patient presenting with a papulopearly BCC. **B** Excision and coverage with an LLL-flap. **C** and **D** At 3 years there has been no recurrence. The result is considered "excellent"; note the symmetry of the nasolabial fold

Fig. 4.7 A–D. Nasolabial fold – kite flaps. **A** In this 64-year-old patient there is sufficient skin laxity to carry out an elliptical excision, but this would lead to asymmetry of the nasolabial folds. **B** Two kite flaps pedicled on subcutaneous fat are approximated. **C** and **D** At 2 years there has been no recurrence. The result is judged "excellent" since the scars are nearly invisible and the nasolabial fold is preserved at rest and during smiling

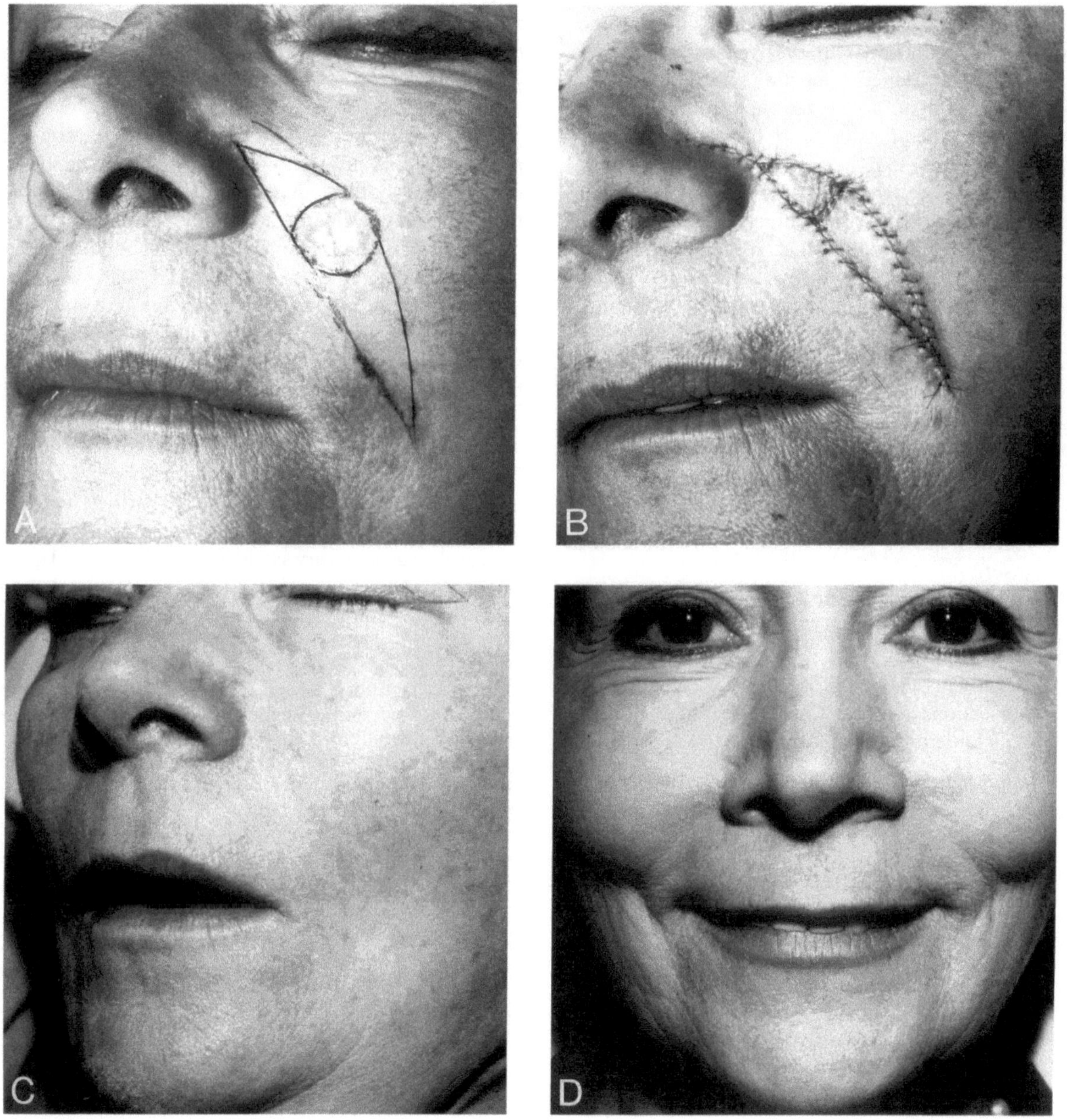
A
B
C
D

The Lips

The contour of this region is complex due to the presence of the philtrum in the upper lip, the overhang in the lower lip, and the mucocutaneous junction which must not be altered. The soft-tissue laxity of the lips promotes permanent deformity when tension is not directed correctly.

Elliptical excision may be considered in the white lip and is oriented radially around the buccal orifice. The defect must be small and sufficiently far from the vermilion border to avoid crossing the mucocutaneous junction. Although the skin is firmly adherent to the m. orbicularis, undermining must be extensive enough to prevent the development of a depressed scar.

Full-thickness wedge resection is frequently indicated in the lip whether the defect involves the vermilion border (rarely for BCCs) or is located nearby (Fig. 4.8). This technique often provides best alternative and avoids secondary deformity of the lip when the following conditions are observed:

- The mucocutaneous junction is carefully tattooed at the outset
- The excision is carried out cleanly with a no. 11 blade
- The muscle layer is sutured and the vermilion border is aligned perfectly
- The excision in the upper lip is limited to 12 mm, since wider resections may result in asymmetry, as illustrated by the patient in Fig. 5.7, p. 94.

Local flaps such as the kite or LLL-flap (Fig. 4.9) are useful for defects that are too large to permit primary closure. Flap design must take into account the location of the beard, although when the defect borders on the beard area or is large one may be obliged to use a flap of hairless skin (Fig. 4.10). When the defect involves the vermilion border, a flap of mucosa may be used along with a skin flap (Color Plate IIC, p. 109).

The philtrum poses a difficult problem because of its precise form. A full-thickness skin graft may be the best solution for defects in this area, although a wedge resection may yield an acceptable result (Fig. 4.11), provided that the outline of the philtral hollow is reconstituted.

A cross-lip or Abbé flap is often the best method to avoid deformity of the upper lip when the defect involves the vermilion border. A wedge resection and primary closure carried out beyond certain limits can distort the philtrum. Therefore, a full-thickness flap is designed on the opposite lip to equal one half the width of the defect. The flap is transferred on the labial artery and carefully inset, while the donor site is closed primarily. The pedicle is divided at 7 days. If the flap has been properly designed the result is usually very satisfactory (Fig. 4.12). The flap has been shown to recover both sensory and motor innervation (Smith 1960).

Fig. 4.8 A–D. Wedge resection of the lip. **A** 60-year-old patient with a BCC of the vermilion border. The mucocutaneous junction is carefully marked. **B** Following wedge resection. **C** A multilayer closure has been carried out including the m. orbicularis. **D** At 6 months the vertical scar is camouflaged by the perioral wrinkles

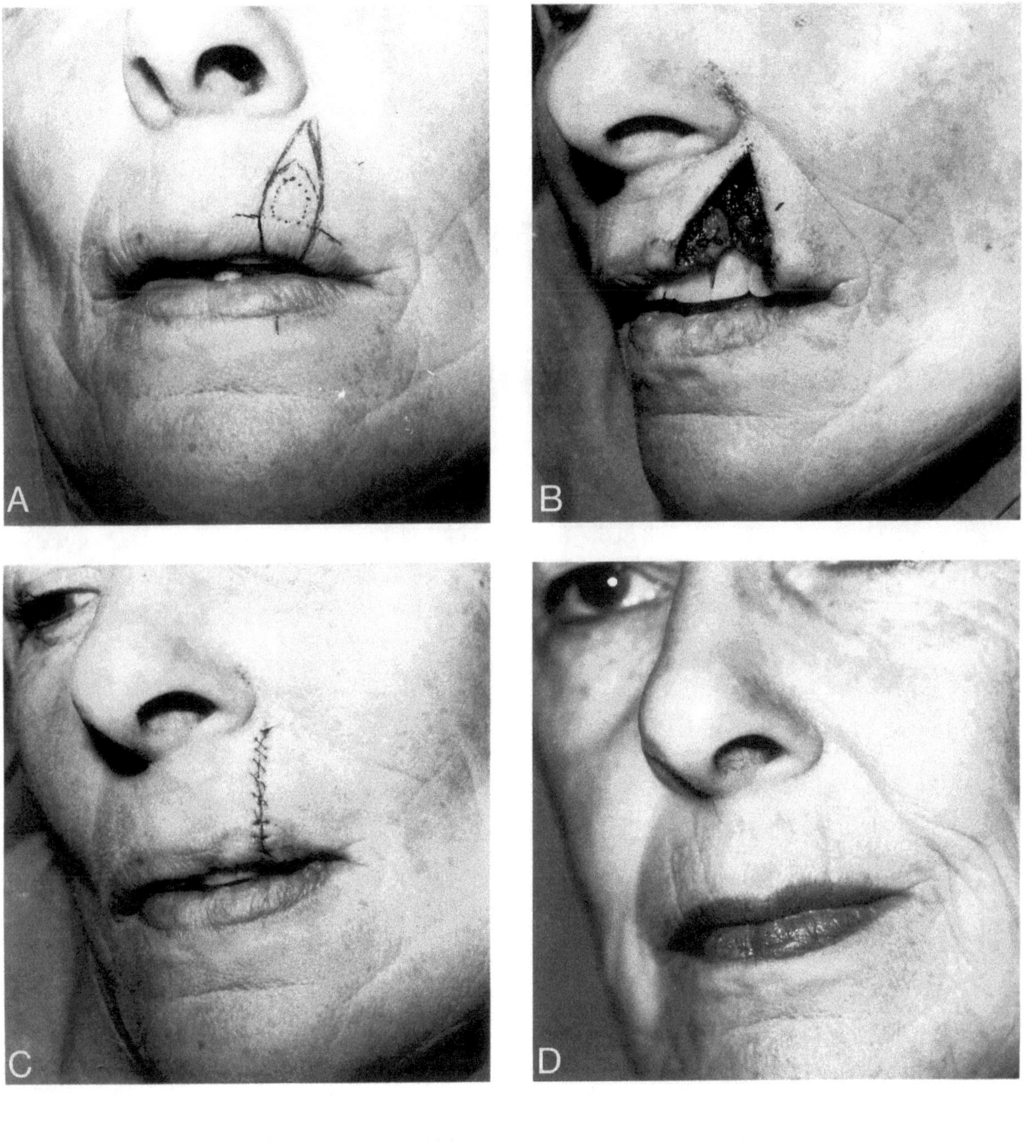
A
B
C
D

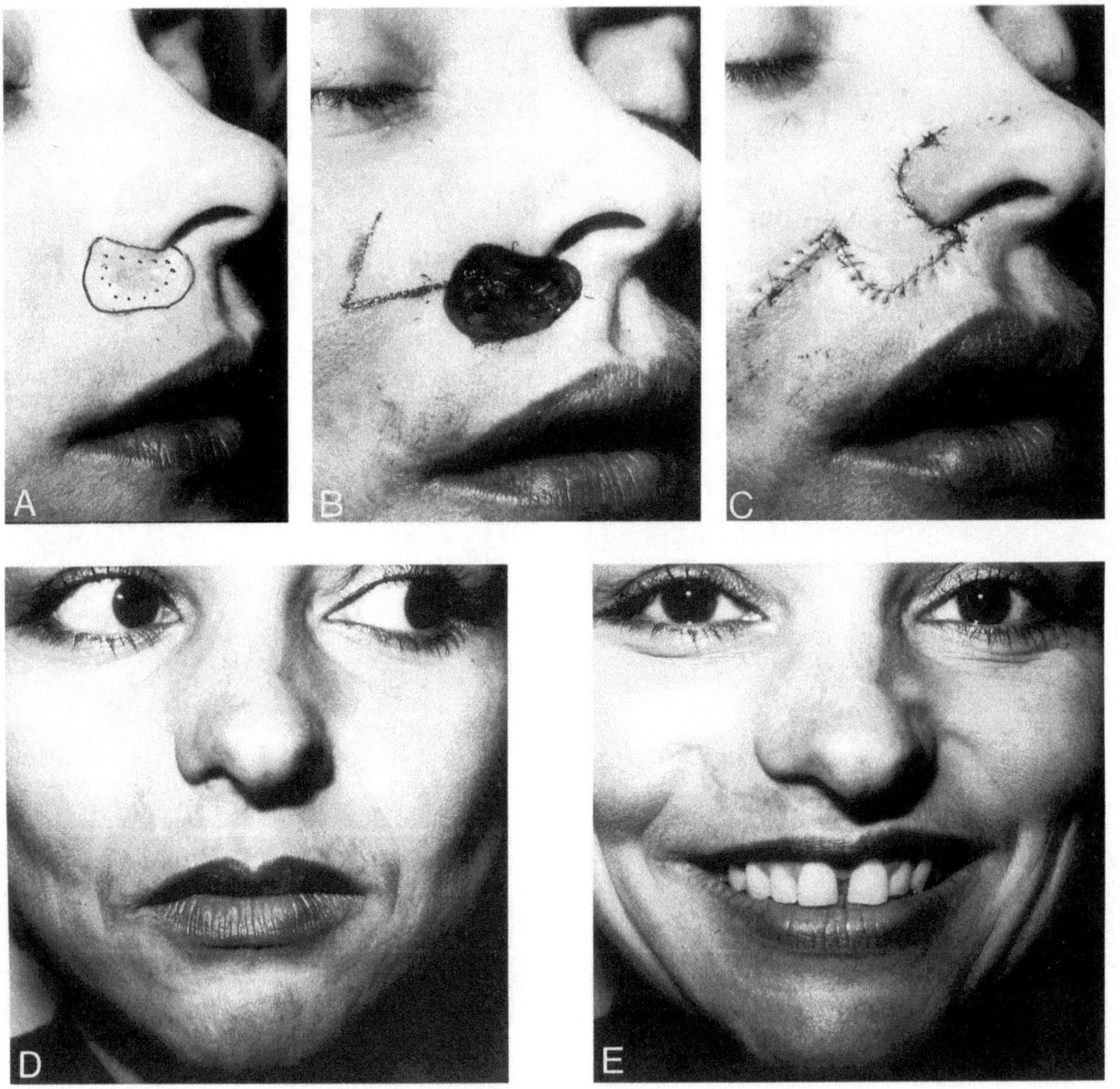

Fig. 4.9 A–E. Upper lip – LLL-flap. **A** 35-year-old patient with a BCC that developed in an old scar. **B** The defect is large and closure must avoid deforming the lip. An LLL-flap is designed to take advantage of skin laxity in the cheek. **C** The excision of the dog-ear created by transposition of the flap is placed along the border of the ala. **D** and **E** At 8 months the appearance at rest is excellent, but during smiling the upper portion of the fold is poorly defined. The result is judged "good"

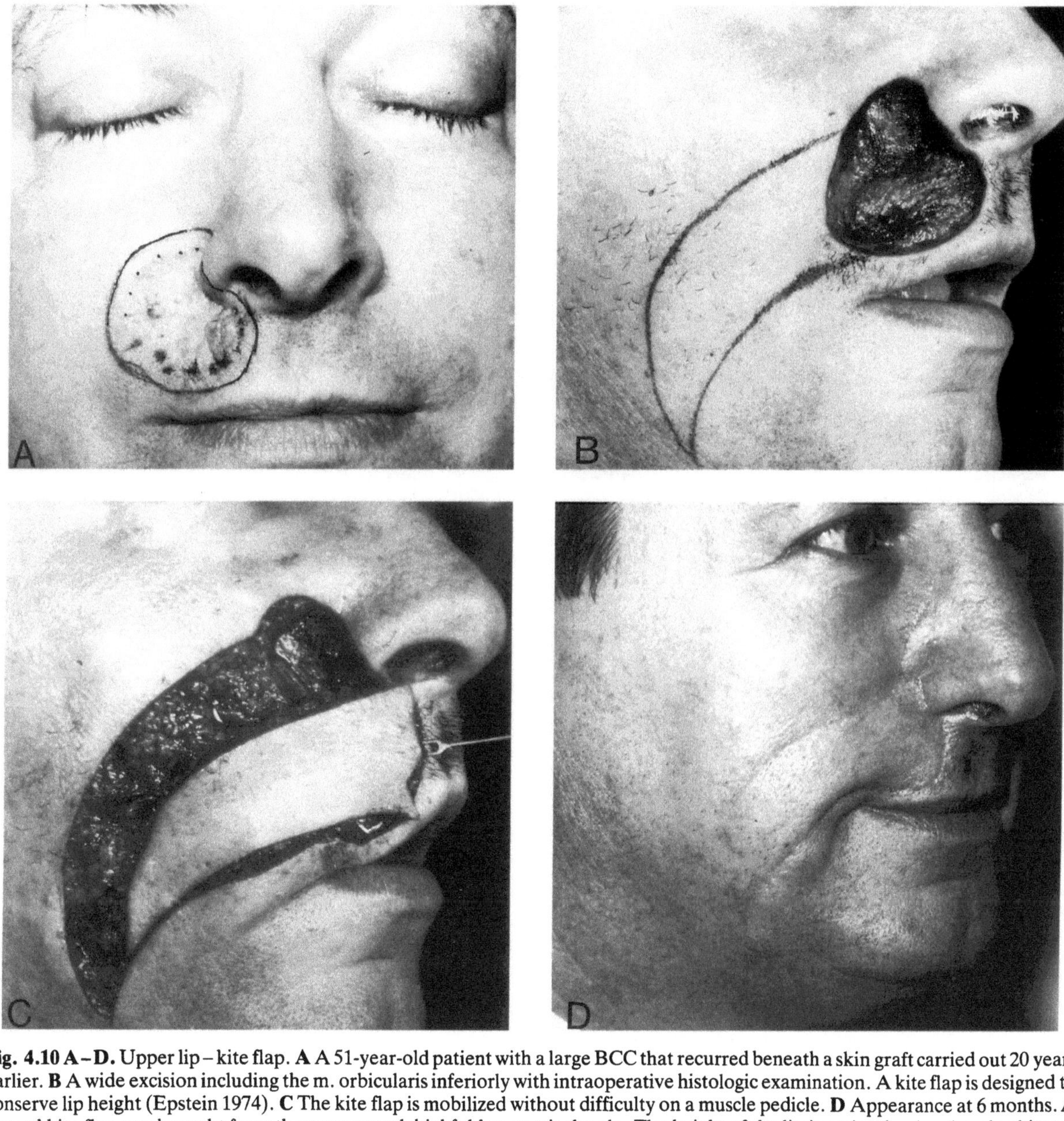

Fig. 4.10 A–D. Upper lip–kite flap. **A** A 51-year-old patient with a large BCC that recurred beneath a skin graft carried out 20 years earlier. **B** A wide excision including the m. orbicularis inferiorly with intraoperative histologic examination. A kite flap is designed to conserve lip height (Epstein 1974). **C** The kite flap is mobilized without difficulty on a muscle pedicle. **D** Appearance at 6 months. A second kite flap was brought from the upper nasolabial fold to repair the ala. The height of the lip is maintained and oral sphincter function is normal. The aesthetic result is judged "mediocre" because the flap is clearly visible, especially since it has brought hairless skin onto the lip

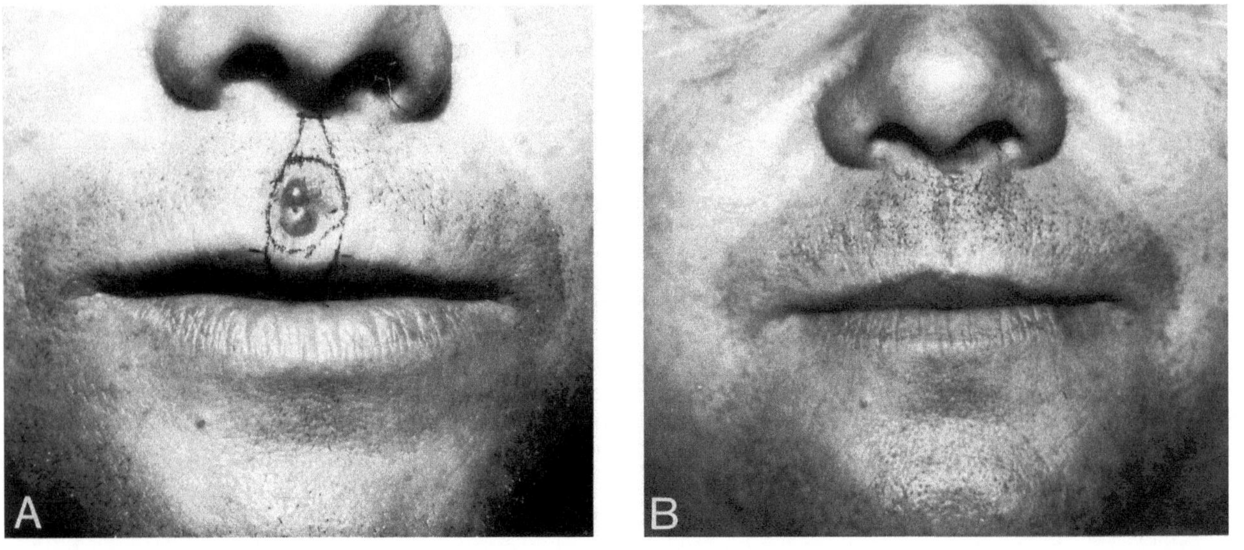

Fig. 4.11 A, B. Philtrum – wedge resection. **A** A BCC of the philtrum in a 45-year-old man. **B** Three months following wedge resection; the Cupid's bow has been lost, but a median depression was created by resecting subcutaneous tissue in the midline

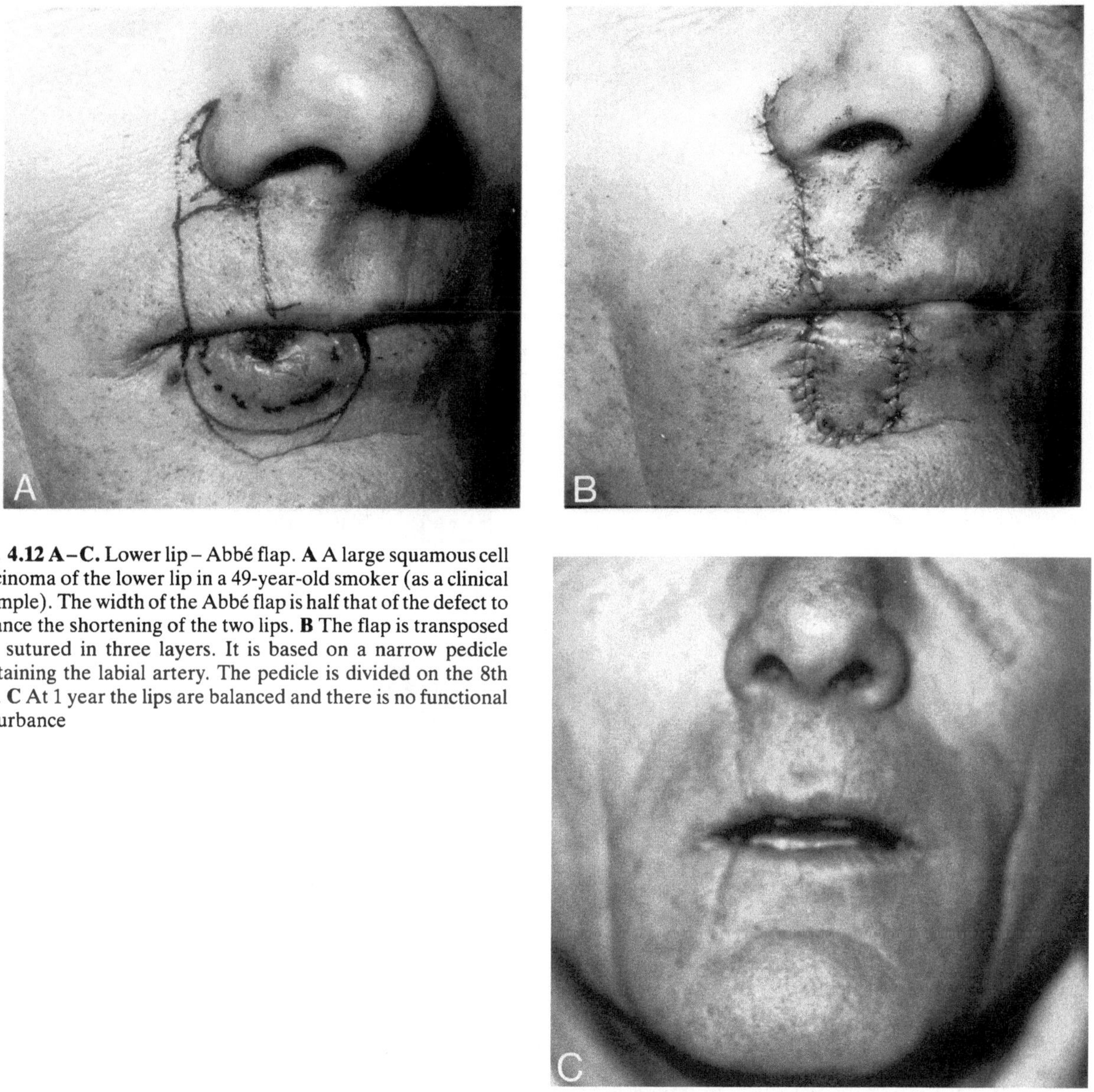

Fig. 4.12 A–C. Lower lip – Abbé flap. **A** A large squamous cell carcinoma of the lower lip in a 49-year-old smoker (as a clinical example). The width of the Abbé flap is half that of the defect to balance the shortening of the two lips. **B** The flap is transposed and sutured in three layers. It is based on a narrow pedicle containing the labial artery. The pedicle is divided on the 8th day. **C** At 1 year the lips are balanced and there is no functional disturbance

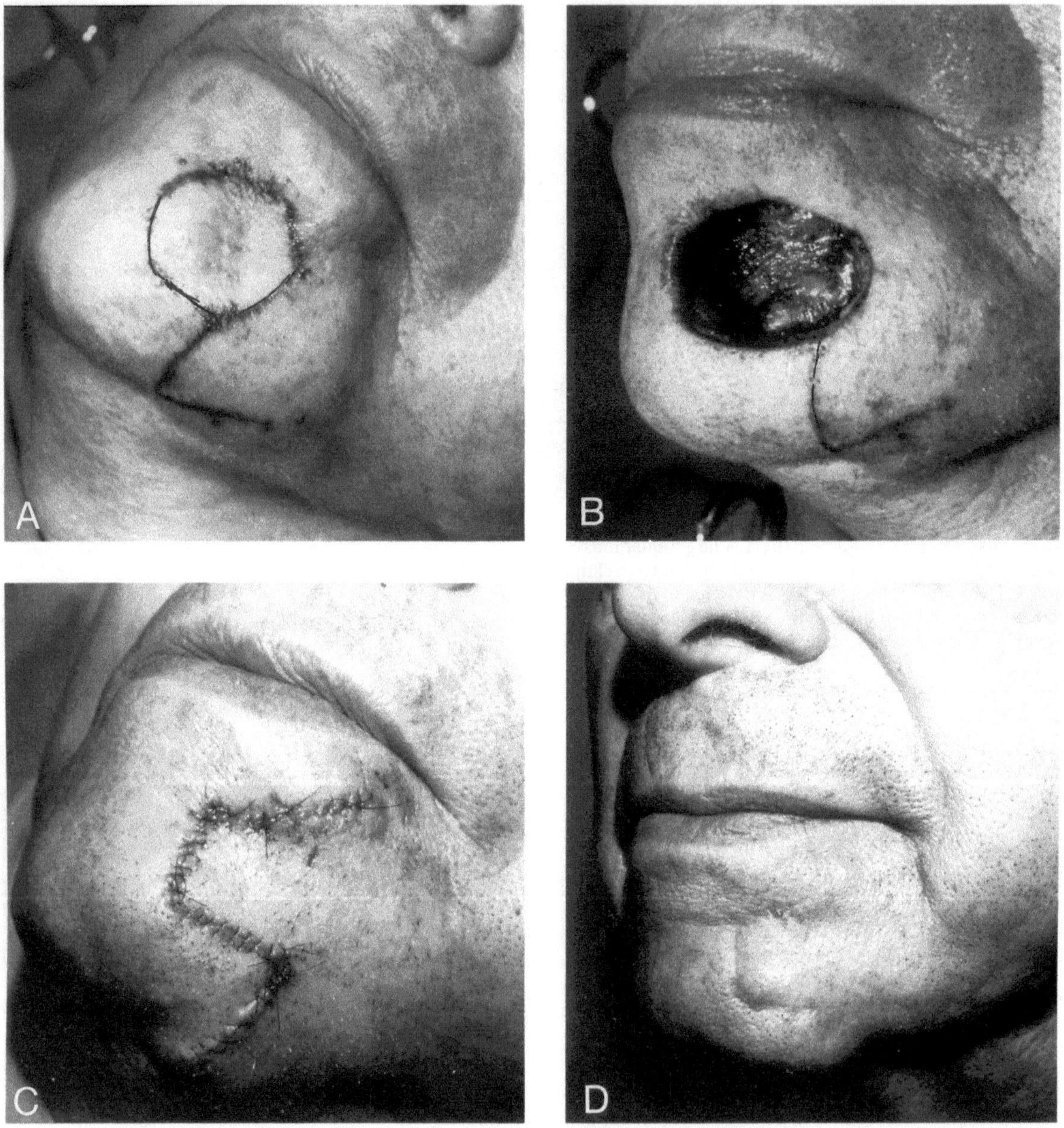
A
B
C
D

The Chin

This area is characterized by significant laxity but its convex contour must not be changed. Accordingly, the elliptical excision is indicated for small repairs, but the LLL-, H- or kite flap must be used when primary closure would produce flattening of the lip (Fig. 4.13).

The Nose

This is a particularly important area because of the frequency of BCCs at this site, the visibility of scarring and other deformities, and the difficulty of repair in this region. Repair is made more difficult by the existence of distinct cutaneous zones over the root of the nose, the middle third, and the tip. The type of skin over the tip is variable; in some cases it is thin enough to transmit the form of the alar cartilages, while in others it is thick and sebaceous. Finally, there is no cutaneous laxity, and furthermore the skin may be tented over a nasal hump.

Elliptical excision and primary closure are therefore rarely indicated. It is sometimes possible to close midline defects with a longitudinal ellipse, although the results may be compromised by an inferior dog-ear which rounds the nasal tip.

Small local flaps such as the LLL- (Fig. 4.14) or kite flap or even bilobed flaps may be used to close small defects up to 8 mm in diameter. Above this limit the tension may be excessive and the frontonasal flap is preferred.

The frontonasal flap (Marchac 1970) was used on 50 occasions in the present series following excisions of BCCs. This is a large rotation flap which takes advantage of the excess skin situated in the glabellar region. The vascular pedicle is well defined and is located in the area of the medial canthus. The narrowness of the pedicle increases the mobility of the flap and allows precise inset into the defect (Fig. 4.15).

The frontonasal flap mobilizes practically all the soft tissue above the defect and provides tension-free coverage with skin that is of the same texture as that to be replaced. The long scar is hidden at the periphery of the nose, and the incisions become practically invisible. This flap is indicated not only for defects of the middle third of the nose (Fig. 4.16), but particularly for the tip as well, where it is essential to avoid distortion (Fig. 4.17 and Color Plate IC, p. 108).

The flap may be readvanced if secondary reexcision becomes necessary. This was the case with a 36-year-old woman in whom a new lesion appeared 5 years following excision of a BCC over the nasal tip (Fig. 4.18).

The wide exposure obtained during the raising of the flap allows modification of the nasal framework. When the resection involves the underlying alar cartilage, the opposite cartilage may be adjusted to restore symmetry. A prominent dorsal hump may be similarly removed under direct vision.

The forehead flap may be necessary in very large resections (Fig. 4.19). When the forehead skin is tight we use a flap of the frontal muscle covered with a full-thickness skin graft, as described by Prof. Song (Song et al. 1982; Fig. 4.20). In certain cases there are indications for the Washio retroauricular flap (see p. 25) or even the Converse scalping flap. These necessitate two stages for division and insetting of the pedicle.

Fig. 4.13 A–D. Lesion of the chin – LLL-flap. **A** A sclerosing BCC that recurred following electrodesiccation in an 81-year-old man. **B** Following a deep excision with intraoperative histology, an LLL-flap is designed to take advantage of local skin laxity. **C** The flap fills the entire depth of the defect. **D** At 3 months the lip is not distorted but there is a mild trapdoor deformity of the flap

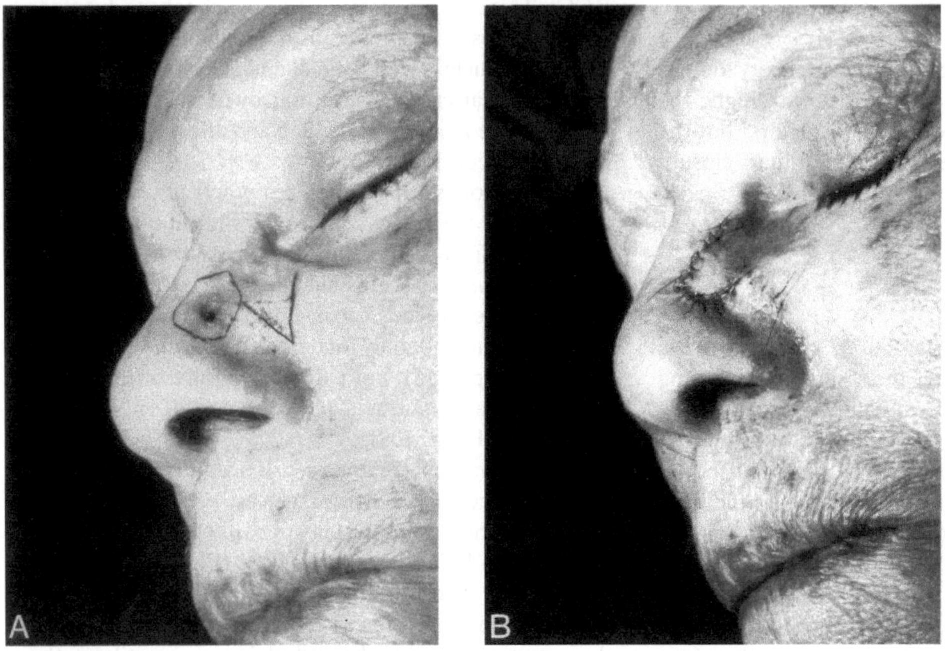

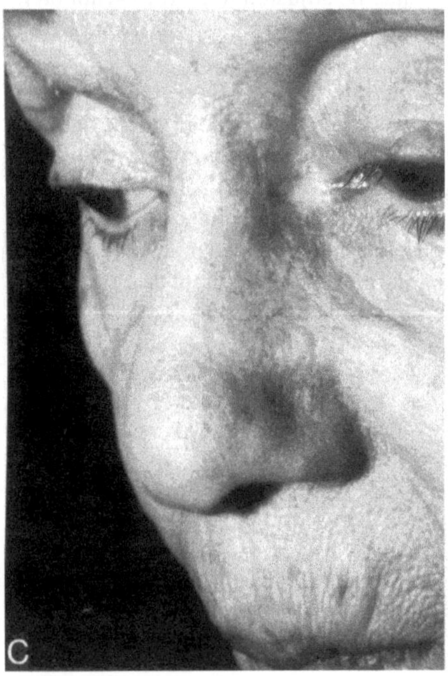

Fig. 4.14 A–C. Small lesion of the nose – LLL-flap. **A** An ulcerated BCC of the nose is an 86-year-old patient. A superior-pedicled LLL-flap is planned. **B** Excess local skin is transposed to the defect. **C** At 6 months the scar is barely visible and there is no deformity. The result is considered “excellent”

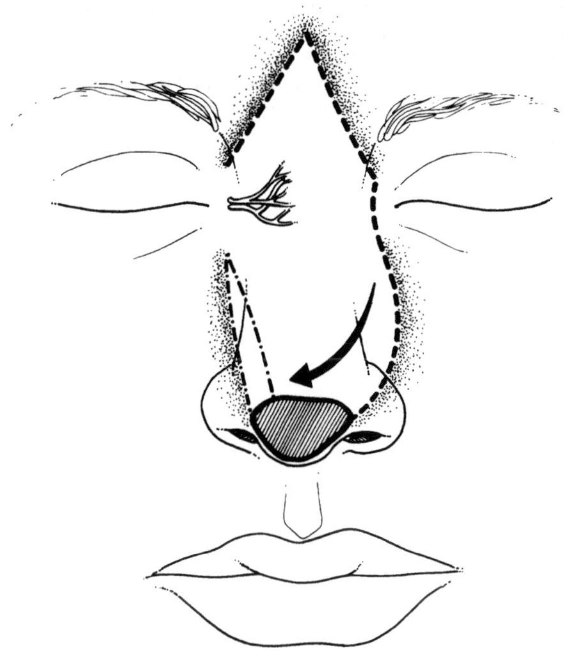

Fig. 4.15. The frontonasal flap (Marchac 1970). The flap is pedicled on the angular vessels and, by mobilizing the entire cutaneous cover of the nose, allows the defect to be filled by an inferior advancement of excess glabellar skin. The pedicle may be extremely narrow, provided it contains the feeding vessels

Finally, the forehead skin can be expanded (Marchac and Larregue 1986) to provide a sizeable flap and still permit primary closure of the donor site (Fig. 4.21).

Full-thickness skin grafts are frequently used in the nose because of their simplicity. However they present two problems:

1. Sucessful take requires the presence of soft tissue over cartilage and bone, but this may have to be sacrificed to provide an adequate excision.
2. The aesthetic result is unpredictable and often mediocre because of differences in thickness, texture, and color between the graft and the skin of the tip.

These problems do not always resolve with time, as illustrated by the young patient shown in Fig. 4.22 and the elderly man in Fig. 4.23. On other occasions, however, the grafts become practically invisible.

The alar region poses difficult problems because of its fineness and delicate modeling. Often, the excision must approach the deep layers to be considered complete. Depending on the location, possible techniques for repair include a full-thickness graft (Fig. 4.24) or a local flap posterior to the defect (Fig. 4.25).

Composite grafts are useful in the reconstruction of the nostril border. They can yield excellent results but may occasionally suffer partial necrosis (Fig. 4.26).

Fig. 4.16 A–D. Dorsum nasi – frontonasal flap. **A** An untreated BCC of the dorsum nasi in a 52-year-old woman. The frontonasal flap extends high onto the forehead. **B** After advancement the tip of the flap has descended to the glabellar region. **C** and **D** At 1 year there is no deformity and the scar is scarcely visible

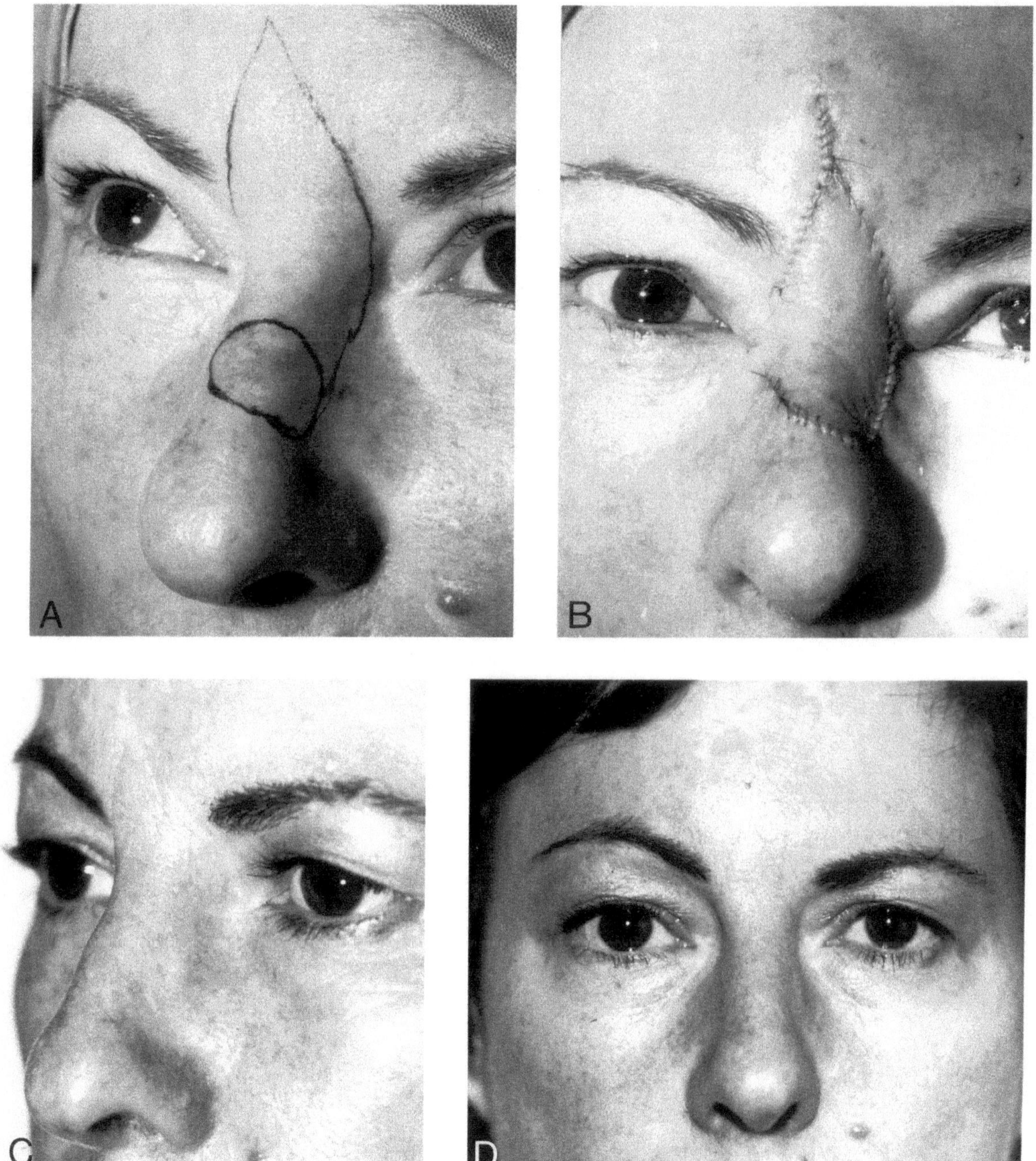
A
B
C
D

Fig. 4.17 A–D. Nasal tip – frontonasal flap. **A** A 70-year-old patient with a BCC of the tip of the nose that developed at the site of an old burn. **B** The excision has exposed the alar cartilages and involves the columella. **C** The frontonasal flap fills the defect without difficulty. **D** At 3 years the aesthetic result is judged "excellent"

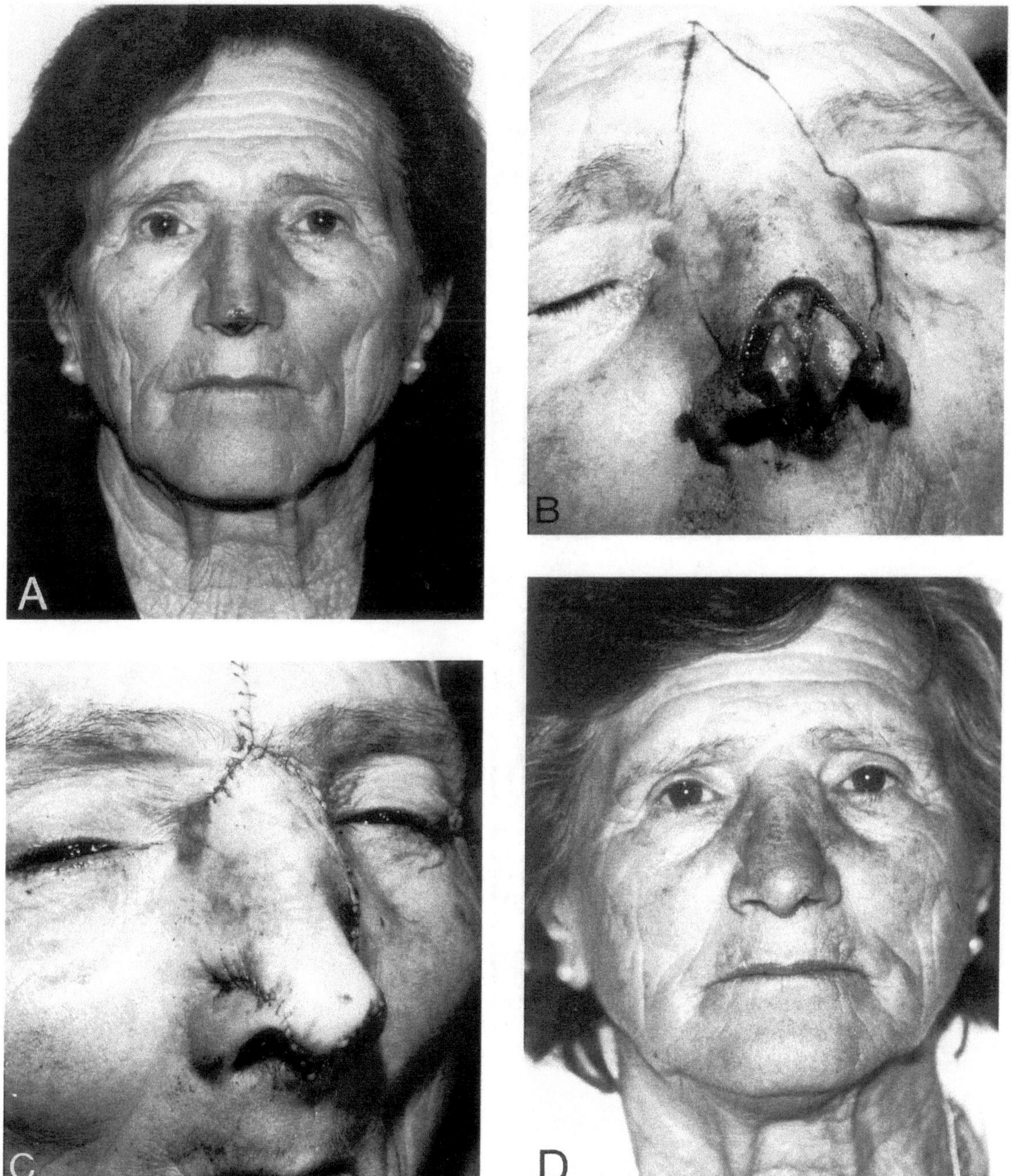
A
B
C
D

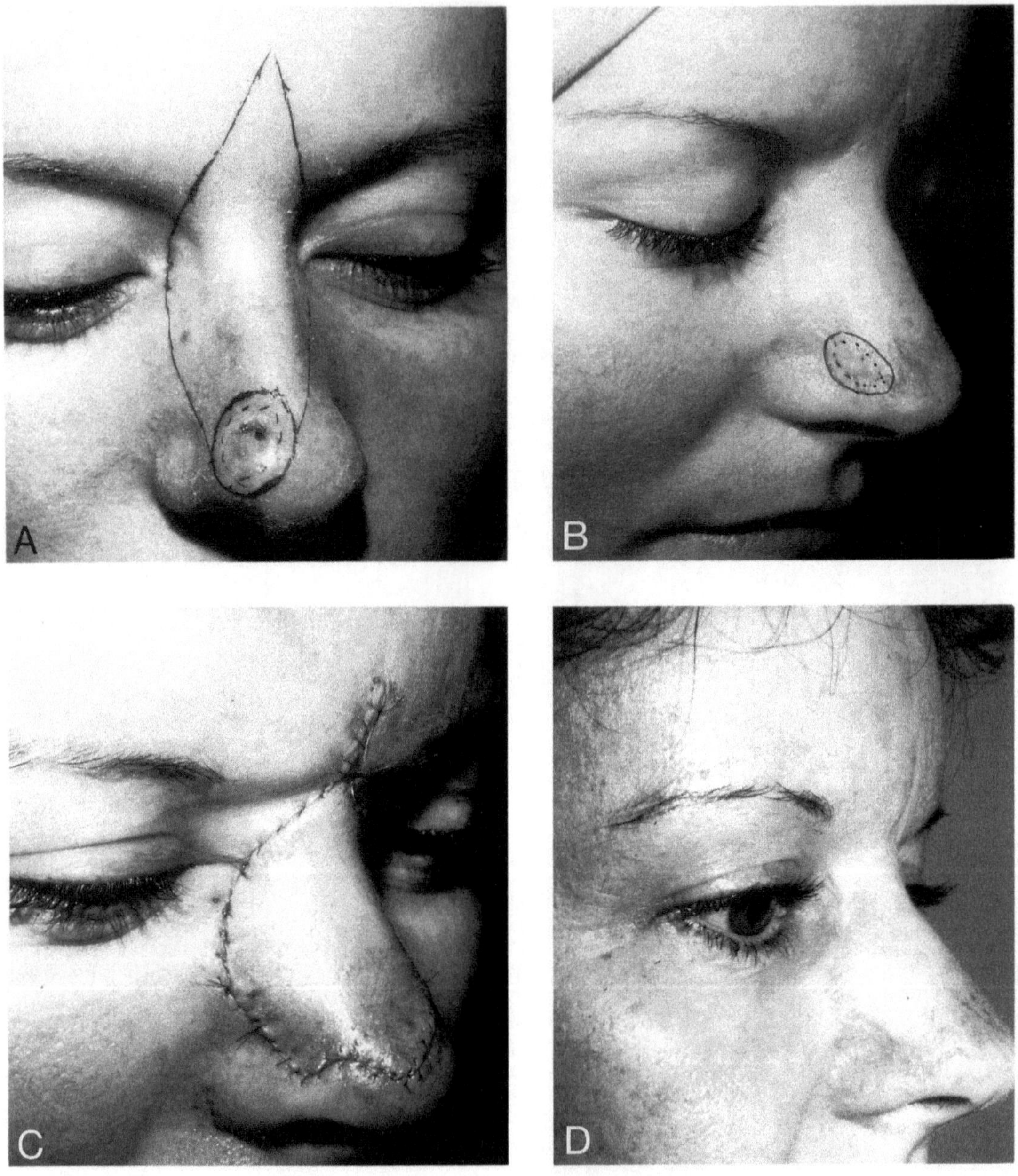

Fig. 4.18 A–D. Nasal tip – frontonasal flap. **A** A 31-year-old patient with a BCC of the right ala. **B** Five years later the lesion has recurred along the border of the flap. **C** After reexcision the flap is readvanced. **D** One year following the second advancement

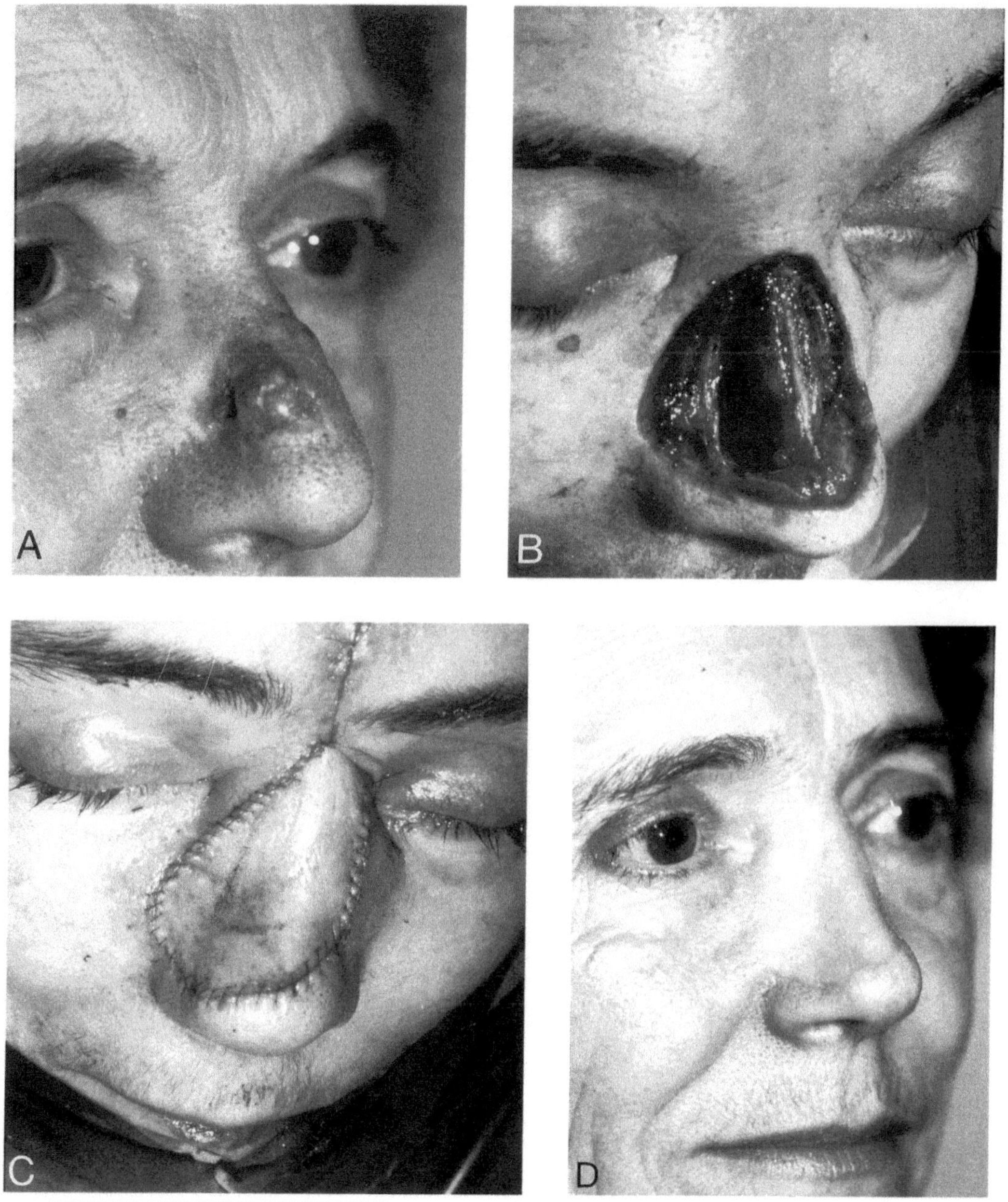

Fig. 4.19 A–D. One-stage forehead flap. **A** This BCC has recurred following radiotherapy in a 57-year-old woman. **B** The full-thickness defect opens into the right nasal fossa. **C** A mucosal flap has provided lining while a midline forehead flap is used to reconstruct the cover. The donor site is closed primarily. **D** At 3 years there is no evidence of recurrence. The aesthetic result is considered only "good" because the scars are visible

Fig. 4.20 A–D. Chinese forehead flap (Song et al. 1982). **A** A new BCC has appeared on the dorsum nasi of a 51-year-old woman who received radiotherapy 10 years earlier. The nasal tip demonstrates the typical appearance of radiodermatitis. **B** The nasal cartilages have been exposed. Because the forehead skin is tight, a flap of the frontal muscle is transposed into the defect. **C** The forehead is closed and a full-thickness graft of retroauricular skin is placed over the muscle. **D** At 6 months the graft take is noted to be poor over the tip

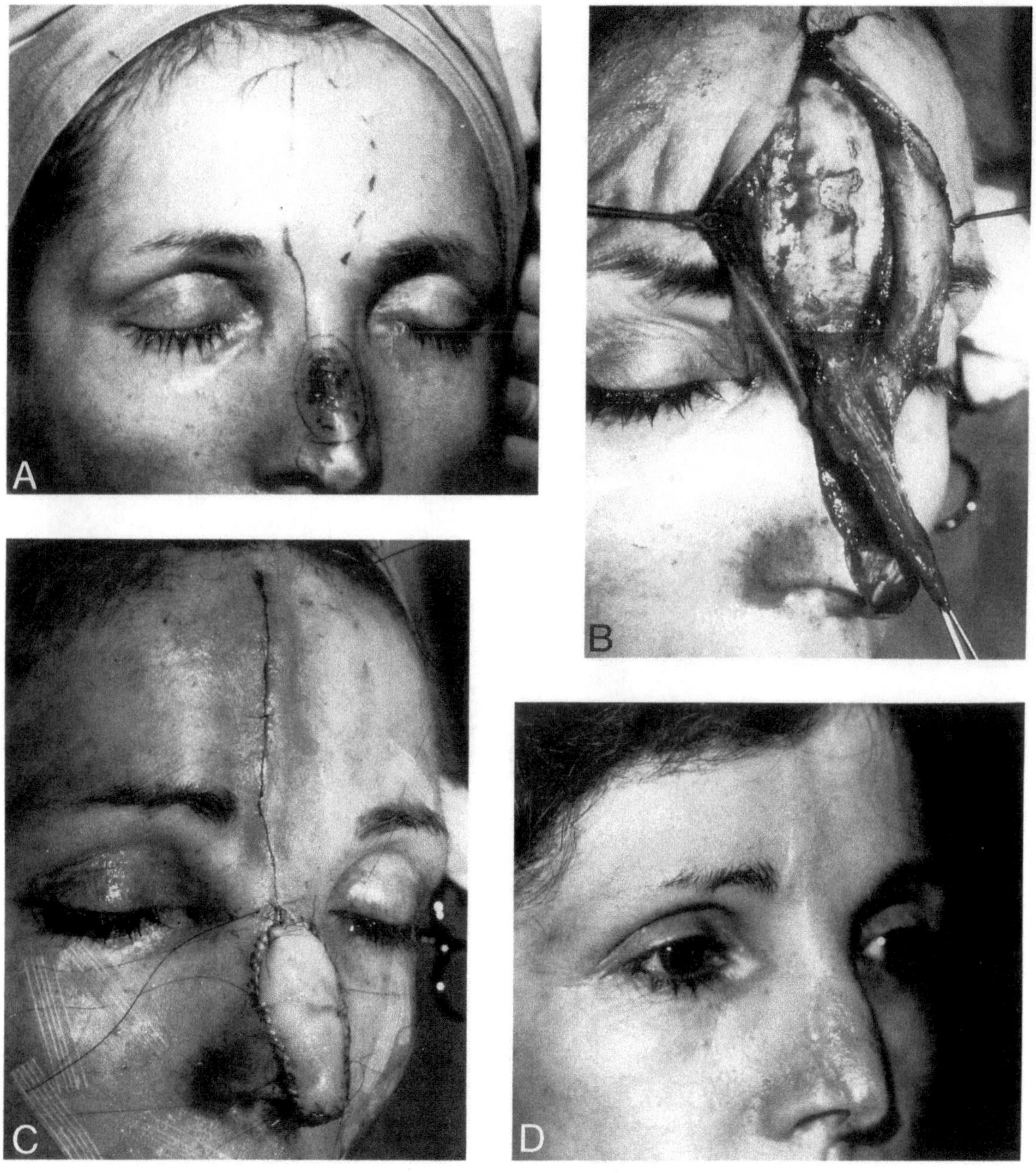
A
B
C
D

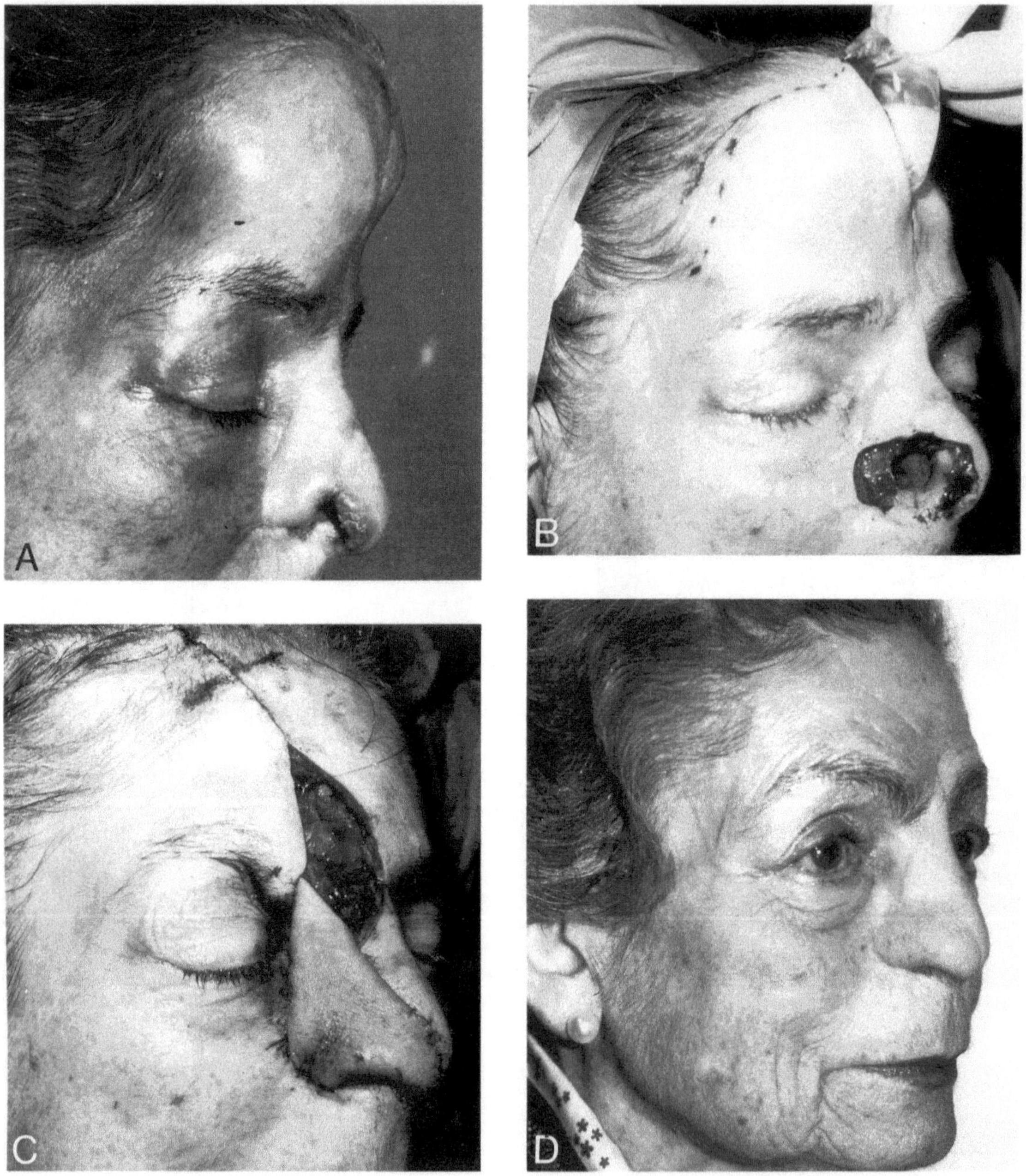
A
B
C
D

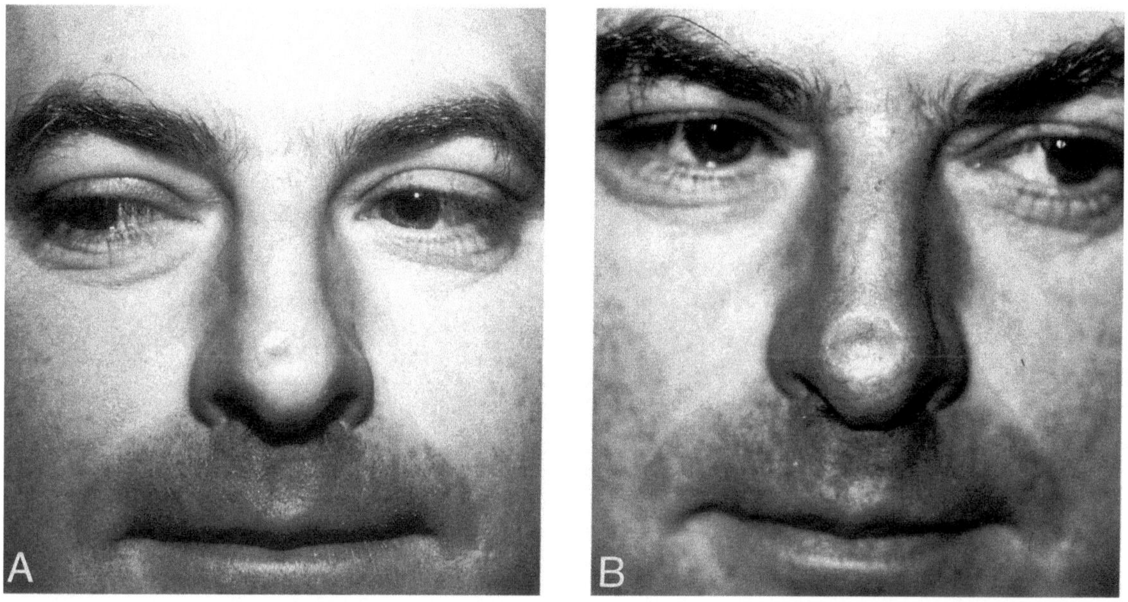

Fig. 4.22 A, B. Full-thickness skin graft. **A** A 37-year-old patient with a primary BCC. **B** Five years after excision and application of a full-thickness skin graft with good take. The patient requested correction of the patchwork appearance

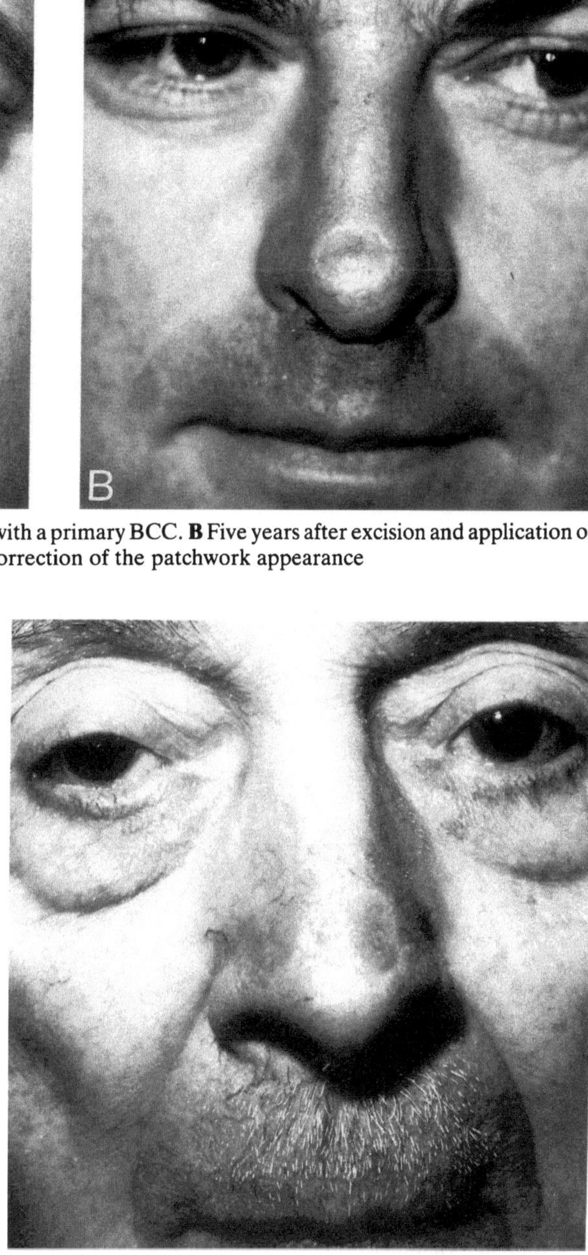

Fig. 4.23. This 92-year-old patient also complained of the patchwork appearance of a skin graft placed 3 years earlier following excision of a BCC of the nasal tip

◀ **Fig. 4.21 A–D.** Expanded forehead flap. **A** This 81-year-old woman presented with the sixth recurrence of a BCC of the right ala. A previous forehead flap had exhausted the forehead laxity, and the patient refused to have the donor site grafted. The slow growth of the tumor permitted us to undertake skin expansion over a period of 6 weeks. **B** The excision has been carried out with intraoperative verification of the margins, and the expander is removed. **C** The flap has been raised and the expanded forehead allows primary closure of the donor site. **D** At 1 year there is minimal deformity of the forehead

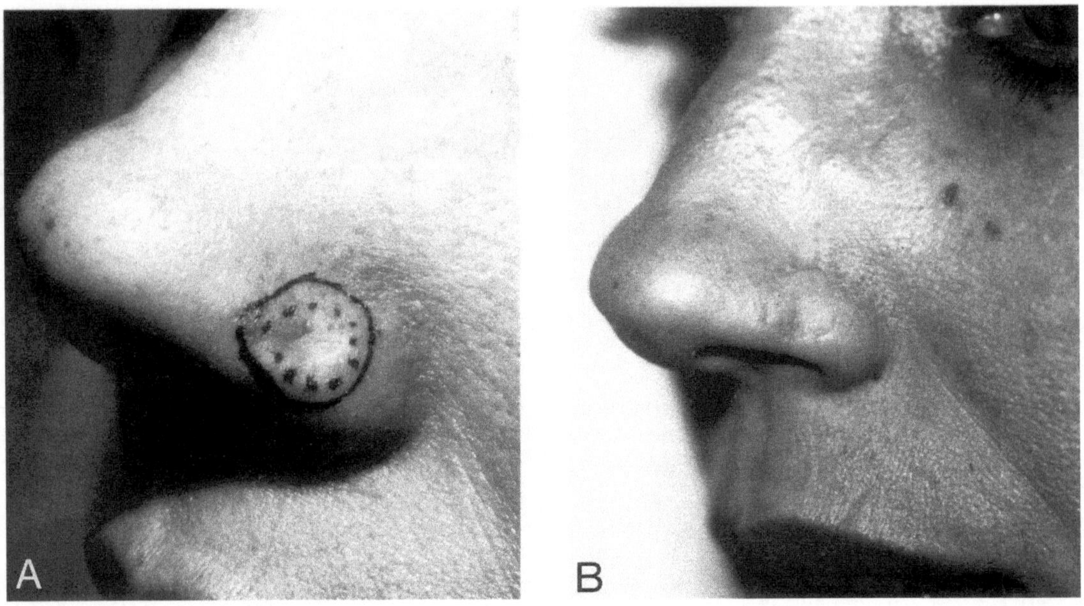

Fig. 4.24 A, B. Ala – full-thickness skin graft. **A** Sclerosing BCC in a 33-year-old woman. **B** One year after repair with a preauricular graft. The result is judged only "good" because although the delicate structure of the ala is preserved, the graft is visible

Fig. 4.25 A–D. Ala – kite flap. **A** This 28-year-old patient presented with a BCC that rapidly recurred following electrodesiccation. **B** A deep excision was carried out, and a kite flap was raised. **C** The flap in place. **D** At 1 year the nasolabial fold is poorly defined but there is no deformity

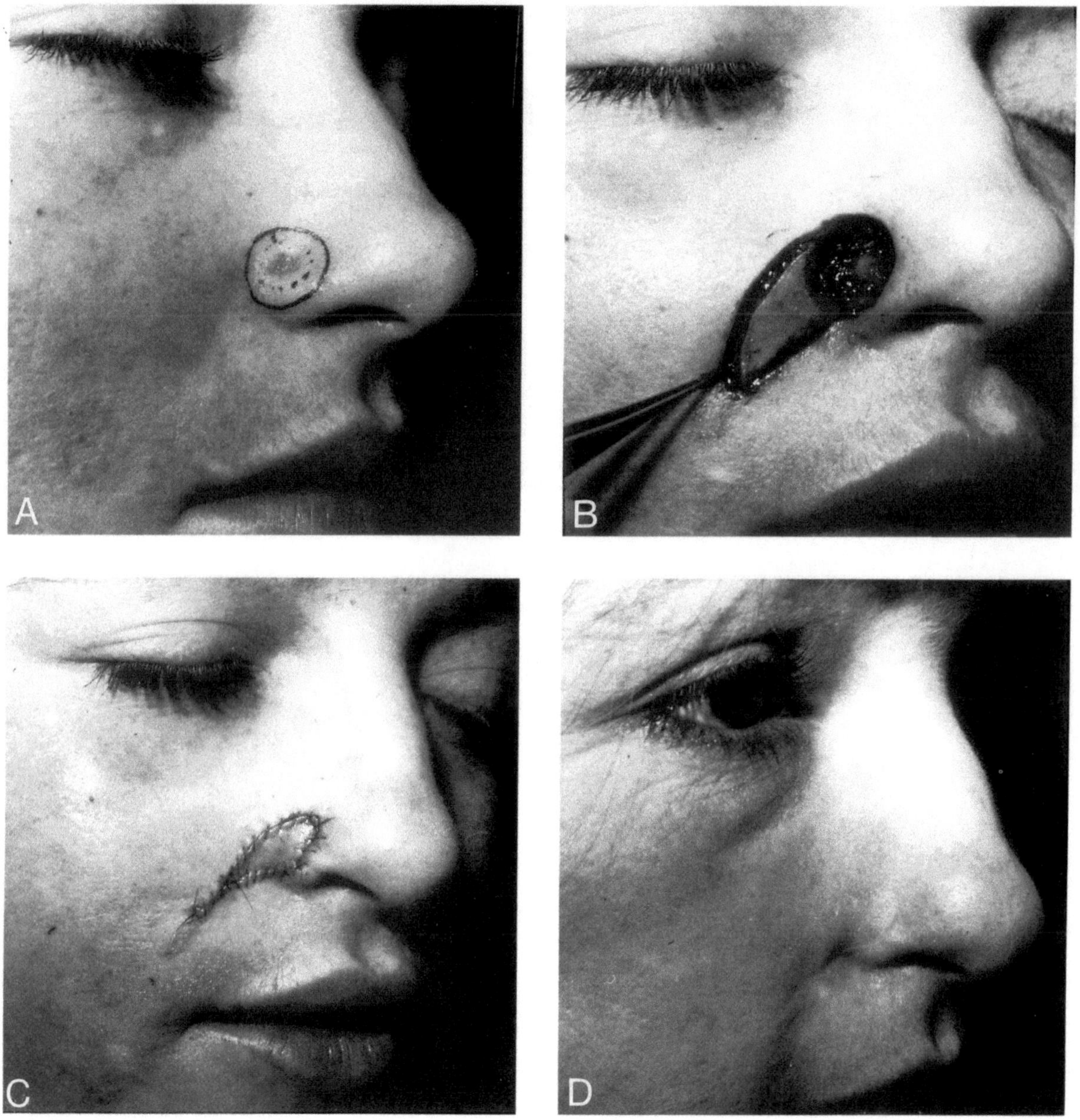
A
B
C
D

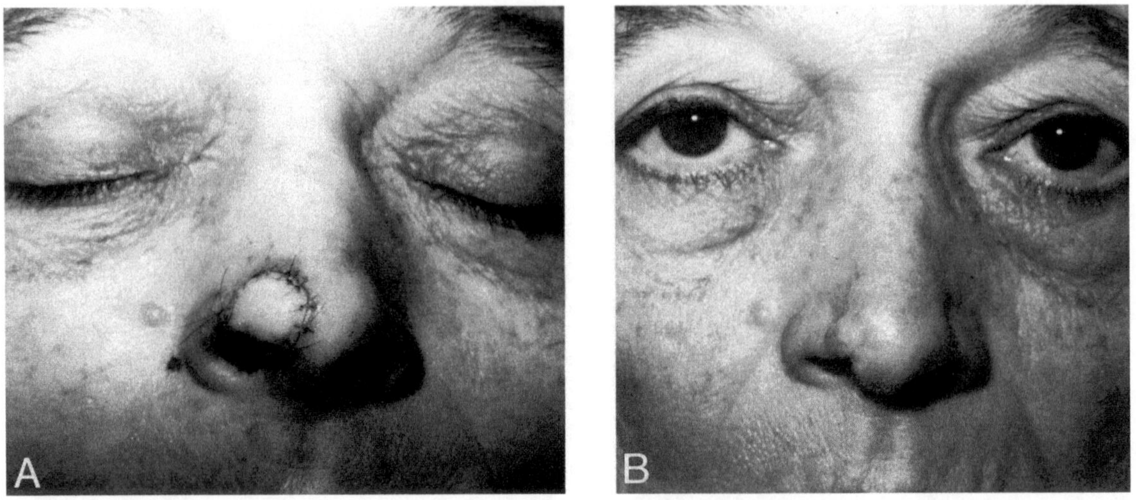

Fig. 4.26 A, B. Composite graft of the ala. **A** A composite graft comprising cartilage and two layers of skin is harvested from the ear to repair a full-thickness alar defect resulting from excision of a BCC. **B** At 1 year a partial loss of the graft has resulted in a small notch

The Eyelids

These are fine, highly mobile structures. The eyelid margin must be preserved or reconstructed and must maintain its normal position. The lacrimal points, especially in the lower lids, and the canthal regions are other problem areas.

The skin of the eyelid is thin, and resection usually includes the m. orbicularis. One must place the eyelid under tension to assess the extent of the defect.

Small lesions may be excised elliptically and closed primarily, with orientation of the ellipse in natural wrinkles or smile lines. With the lower lid, care must be taken to verify that the lid margin is not abnormally depressed when the patient looks upward. Otherwise, one runs the risk of producing lagophthalmos (abnormal shortness of the lid) or even ectropion (eversion of the lid) (see Fig. 7.1, p. 105).

When the ellipse is situated in the inferior portion of the lower lid it is advisable to try to follow the border between the lid and the cheek, as the color and texture of the skin change from one region to the other.

In the upper lid one can often carry out large elliptical resections. The ellipse corresponds to that used in aesthetic blepharoplasty. To avoid asymmetry the contralateral lid may be treated similarly (Fig. 4.27).

Frequently, one must use a flap to maintain height, especially in the lower lid. The kite flap allows advancement of excess skin that is always present over the malar prominence and provides excellent results. The blood supply is assured by the m. orbicularis, on which the flap is based (Fig. 4.28 and Color Plate IIB, p. 109). This flap is equally useful in the superior portion of the upper lid (Fig. 4.29), where the elliptical excision is contraindicated as it advances thin skin up to the eyebrow, and modifies the normal bulging of the upper area of the lid. Two kite flaps may be used to maintain the height of the lid.

Use of the forehead flap should be avoided, as it introduces thick skin which is a poor match for the normal eyelid (Fig. 5.6, p. 93). It is inadvisable to use flaps of cheek skin for the same reason. On the other hand, a laterally based flap may be transposed from the upper to the lower lid. This myocutaneous flap is based on the m. orbicularis and utilizes the redundant tissue usually found in the upper lid (Fig. 4.30).

A full-thickness skin graft is indicated when a large area is to be covered. A retroauricular graft can provide a satisfactory result with time (Fig. 4.31). Ideally, the lower lid is resurfaced with skin from one or both upper lids.

We do not believe that the excision should be extended to include the whole lid as is indicated in the repair of burn ectropion. It is sufficient to cover only the defect itself using thin skin.

When *the lid margin* is involved with a BCC a wedge excision is possible, involving up to one third of the width of the lid. The repair must be meticulously carried out in layers, including the tarsoconjunctival layer, the m. orbicularis, and the skin. Identification and perfect apposition of the border of the eyelid will prevent functional and aesthetic complications (Fig. 4.32).

When the resection exceeds one third of the width of the eyelid other procedures are indicated. The lower lid may be reconstructed with a cheek-advancement flap that is lined with a mucocartilaginous graft from the nasal septum or a composite graft from the ear (Fig. 4.33). Techniques used to reconstruct the upper lid include the composite eyelid graft, the combination of a tarsoconjunctival flap and a muscle flap covered with a skin graft, and a switch flap from the lower to the upper lid with the lower lid reconstructed in turn by a cheek-advancement flap (Mustardé 1966).

Situated at the junction of the eyelids and the nose, *the medial canthal area* is of particular interest because of the considerable local frequency of BCCs and the difficulty of excision and repair. The lesion is often situated close to the caruncle and lacrimal points and the deep margin may involve the canthal ligament and the angular vein.

The excision must be designed to provide the necessary margins, without regard for adjacent structures. A fine suction cannula is essential to clear the operative field and allow precise control of the resection. The excision must be radical since recurrence may present grave problems, such as deep extension into the orbit and ethmoid region. One should not hesitate to remove the periosteum and the anterior part of the canthal ligament, as deep invasion is often rapidly attained in this area of very thin skin.

Repair may be carried out by mobilizing local tissues or by full-thickness skin graft when the wound bed is even and well vascularized. Such grafts often provide good results in this area, especially when the residual tissues overlying the bone are very thin. The most useful local flap is Mustardé's glabellar V-Y advancement flap (Fig. 4.34). Occasionally, one can use a kite flap from the upper nasolabial fold or a combination of flaps.

Sacrifice of a lacrimal point presents a number of difficult problems, since reconstruction of the lacrimal canal with vein or arterial grafts is often disappointing. The inferior canaliculus is functionally the more important. If the point must be sacrificed, the end cut can be anastomosed to the conjunctival sac and a catheter left in place for 3 weeks (Color Plate IIA, p. 109). Failure of this procedure or complete sacrifice of the inferior canaliculus may necessitate permanent drainage with a glass or silicone tube into the nasal fossa.

Reconstruction of the *lateral canthal area* is difficult because it requires restoration of the conjunctiva, canthal ligament, and skin (Fig. 4.35).

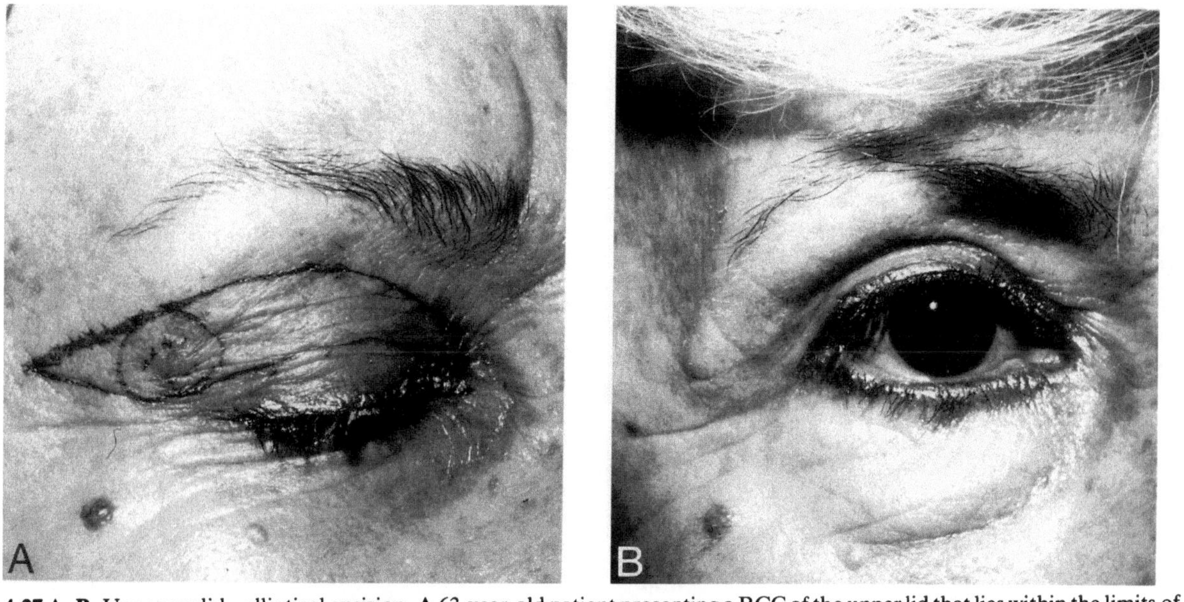

Fig. 4.27 A, B. Upper eyelid – elliptical excision. **A** 63-year-old patient presenting a BCC of the upper lid that lies within the limits of the customary blepharoplasty excision. **B** Four months later the result is satisfactory. A blepharoplasty has to be carried out on the contralateral lid to maintain symmetry

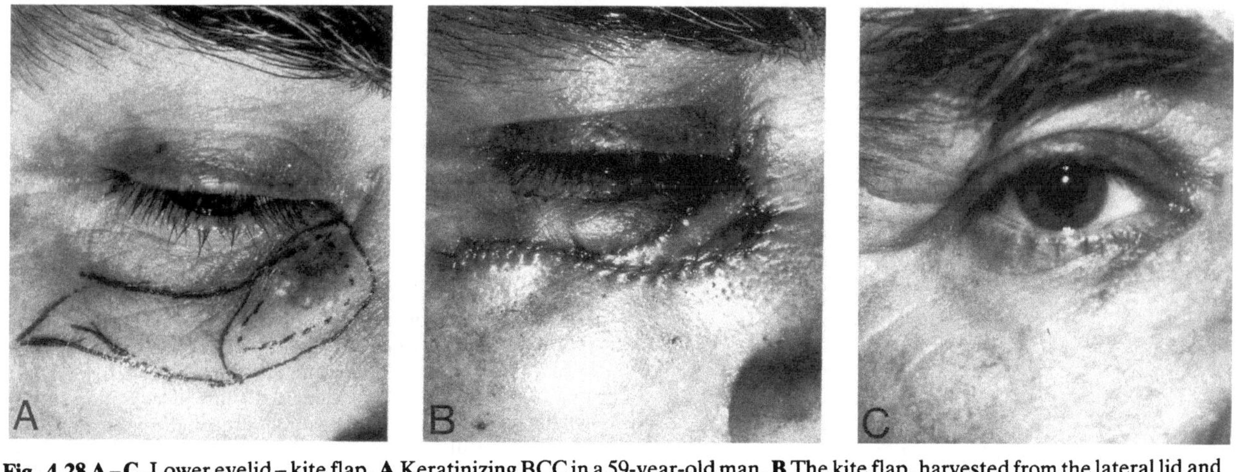

Fig. 4.28 A–C. Lower eyelid – kite flap. **A** Keratinizing BCC in a 59-year-old man. **B** The kite flap, harvested from the lateral lid and based on the m. orbicularis, is advanced easily into the defect. **C** At 10 months the scar is nearly invisible and there is no deformity

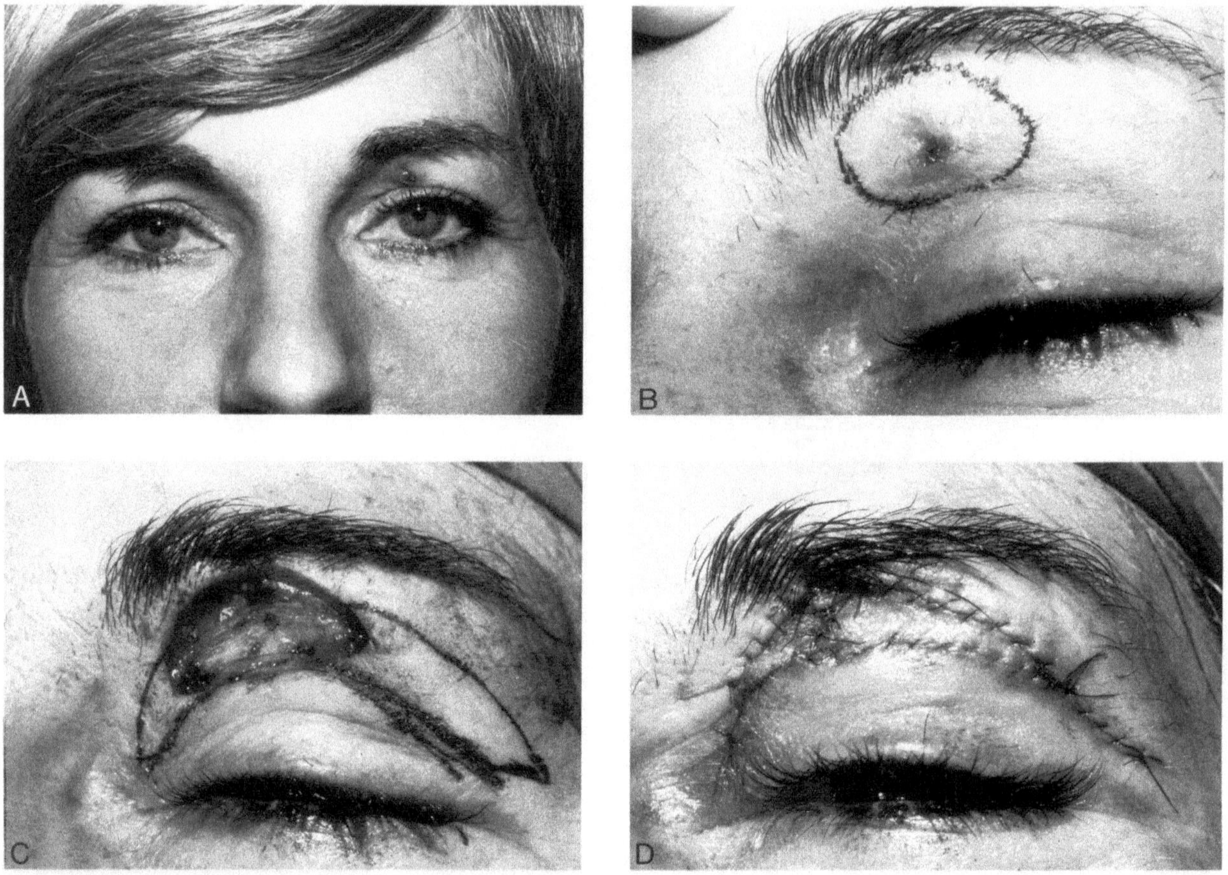

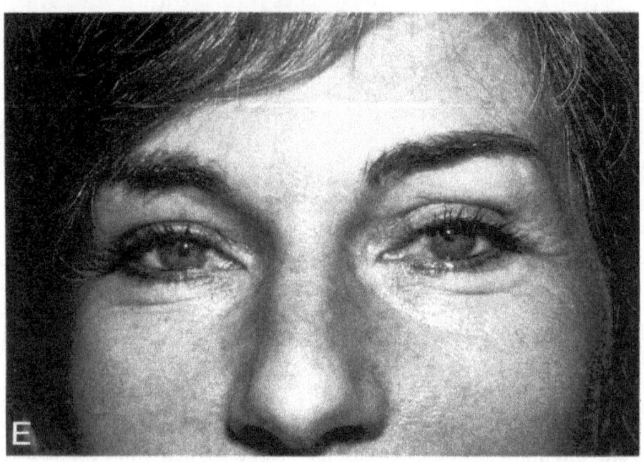

Fig. 4.29 A–E. Upper eyelid – double kite flap. **A** and **B** A 45-year-old woman with an ulcerated BCC of the upper lid. **C** and **D** Elliptical excision would bring the thin palpebral skin into an area of thicker skin. Two kite flaps allow preservation of the height and skin characteristics of this area of the upper lid. **E** At 2 years the result is judged "excellent". There is no deformity or asymmetry and no visible scar

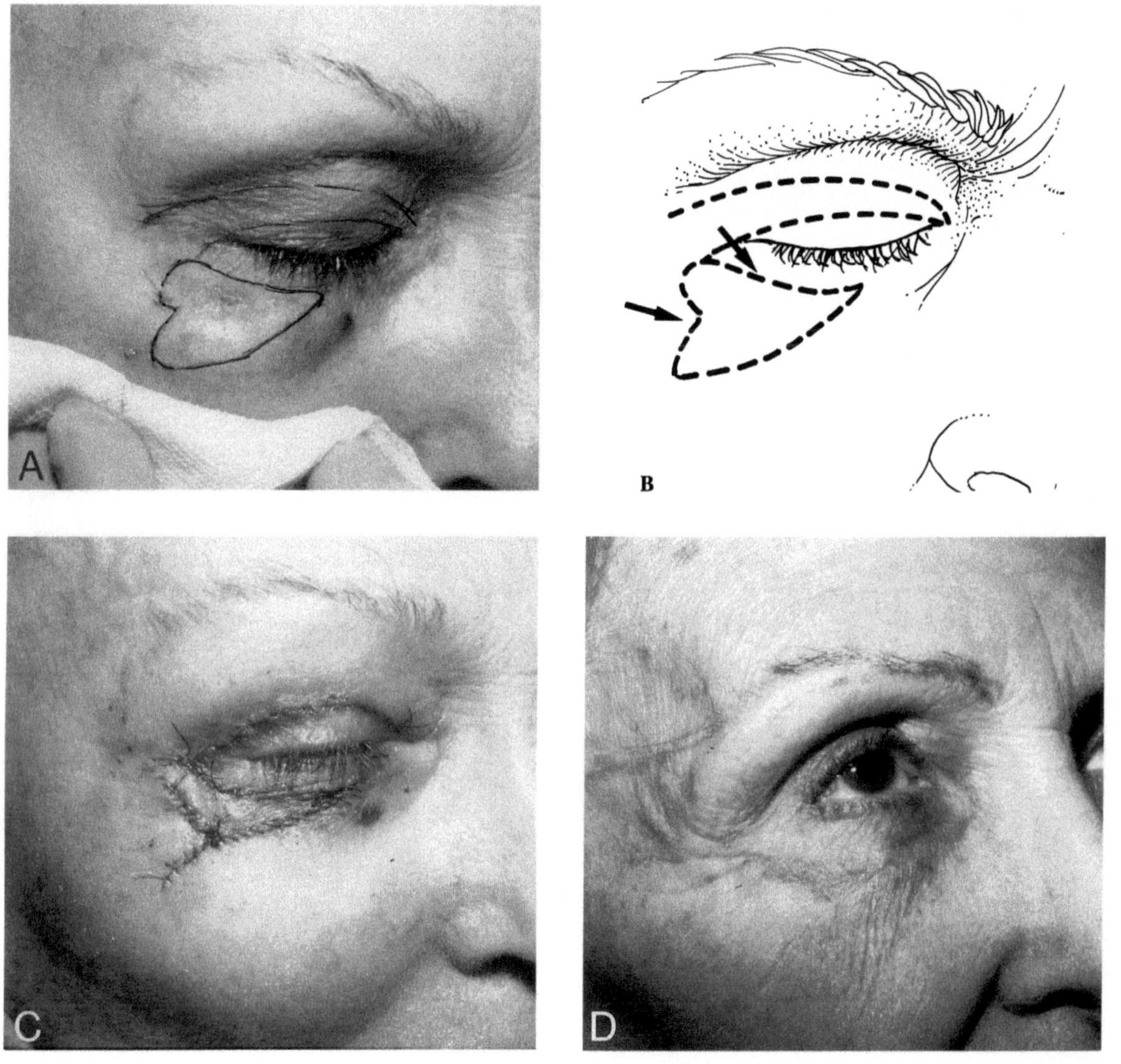

Fig. 4.30 A–D. Lower eyelid – upper lid transposition flap. **A** A large plaque of BCC in the lower lid of a 78-year-old woman. The lesion has recurred following electrodesiccation. **B** Repair combines advancement of the premalar skin with a laterally based transposition flap from the upper lid. **C** The flap in place. **D** At 2 years there is no deformity but the outlines of the flap are visible. The result is considered "good"

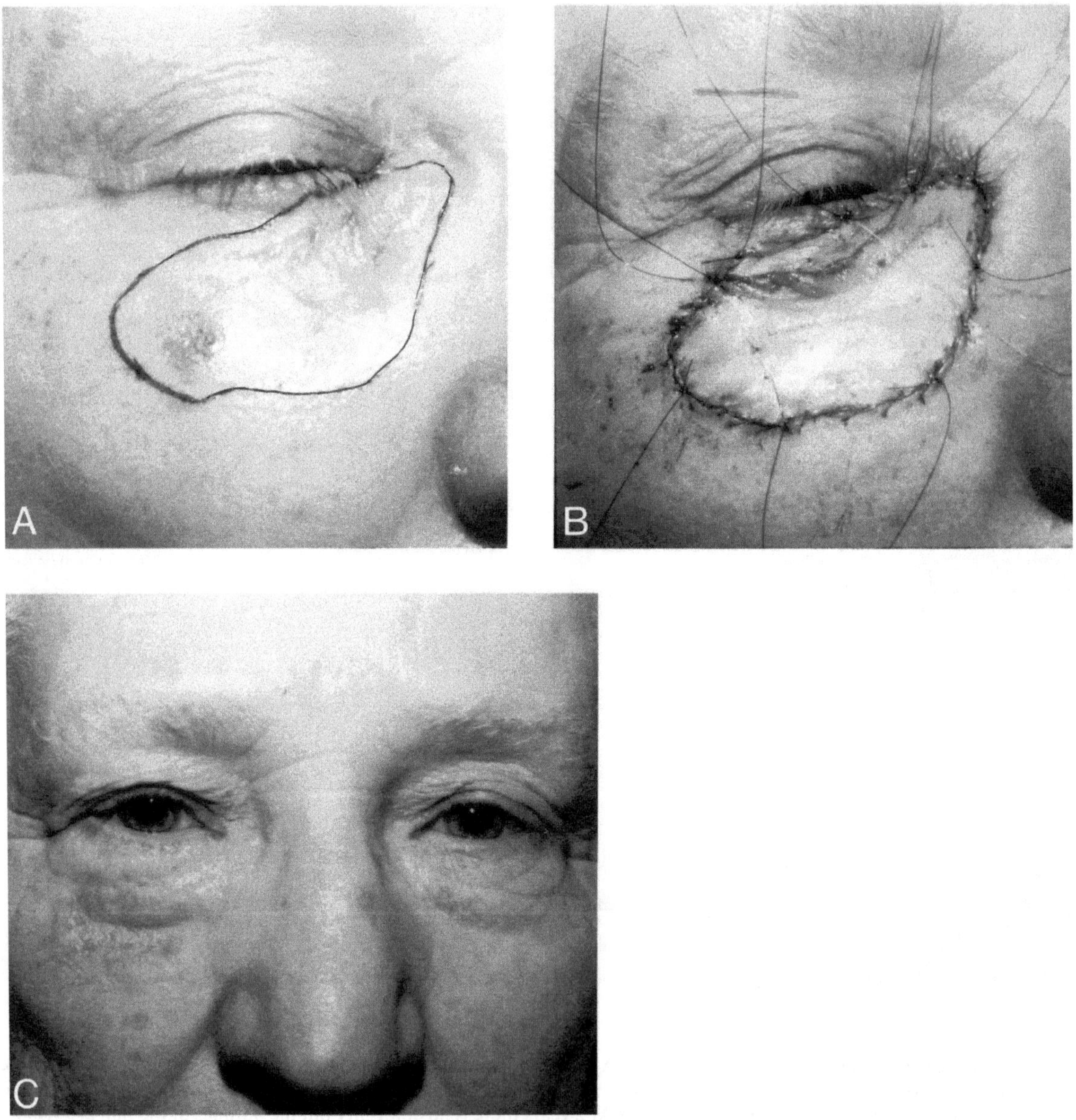

Fig. 4.31 A–C. Lower lid – full-thickness graft. **A** A large plaque of BCC in a 69-year-old woman. **B** Repair with a graft of retroauricular skin. **C** At 1 year the aesthetic result is "excellent" since there is no asymmetry, the skin texture is satisfactory, and the pouches of fat have reappeared

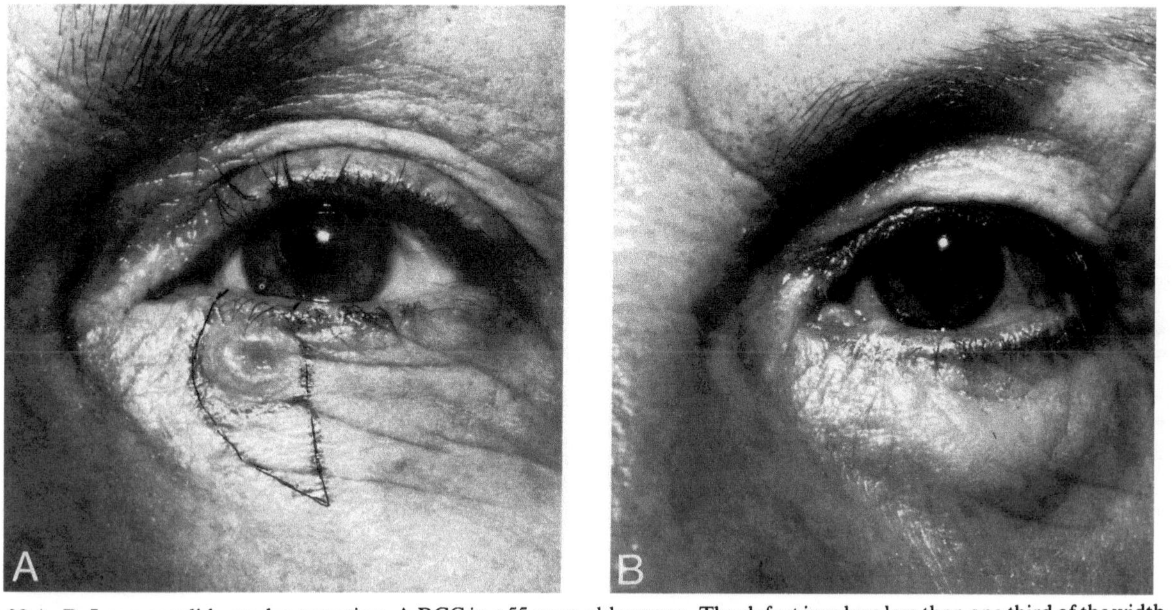

Fig. 4.32 A, B. Lower eyelid – wedge resection. **A** BCC in a 55-year-old woman. The defect involves less than one third of the width of the lid, and primary closure is possible. **B** At 8 years the aesthetic result is "excellent".

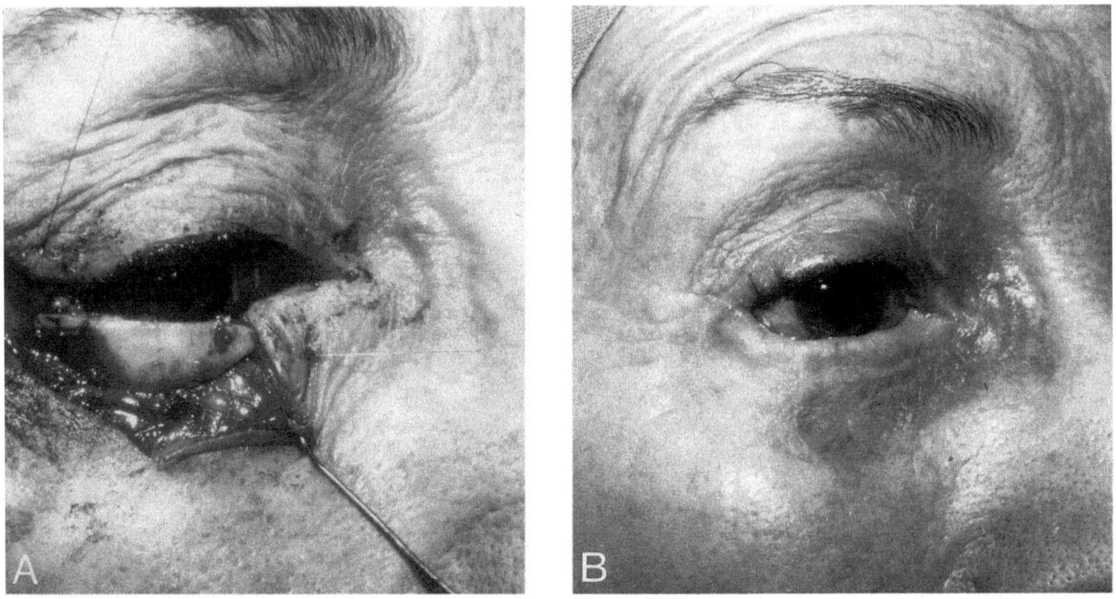

Fig. 4.33 A, B. Lower-eyelid – chondrocutaneous graft. **A** The lateral two thirds of the lower lid were removed in this 64-year-old woman with a twice-recurrent BCC. A chondrocutaneous graft harvested from the concha of the ear supplied lining and support, while cover was provided by a Mustardé-type cheek rotation flap (see Fig. 6.1). **B** At 10 months the position of the lid is acceptable but the overall appearance is not very satisfactory

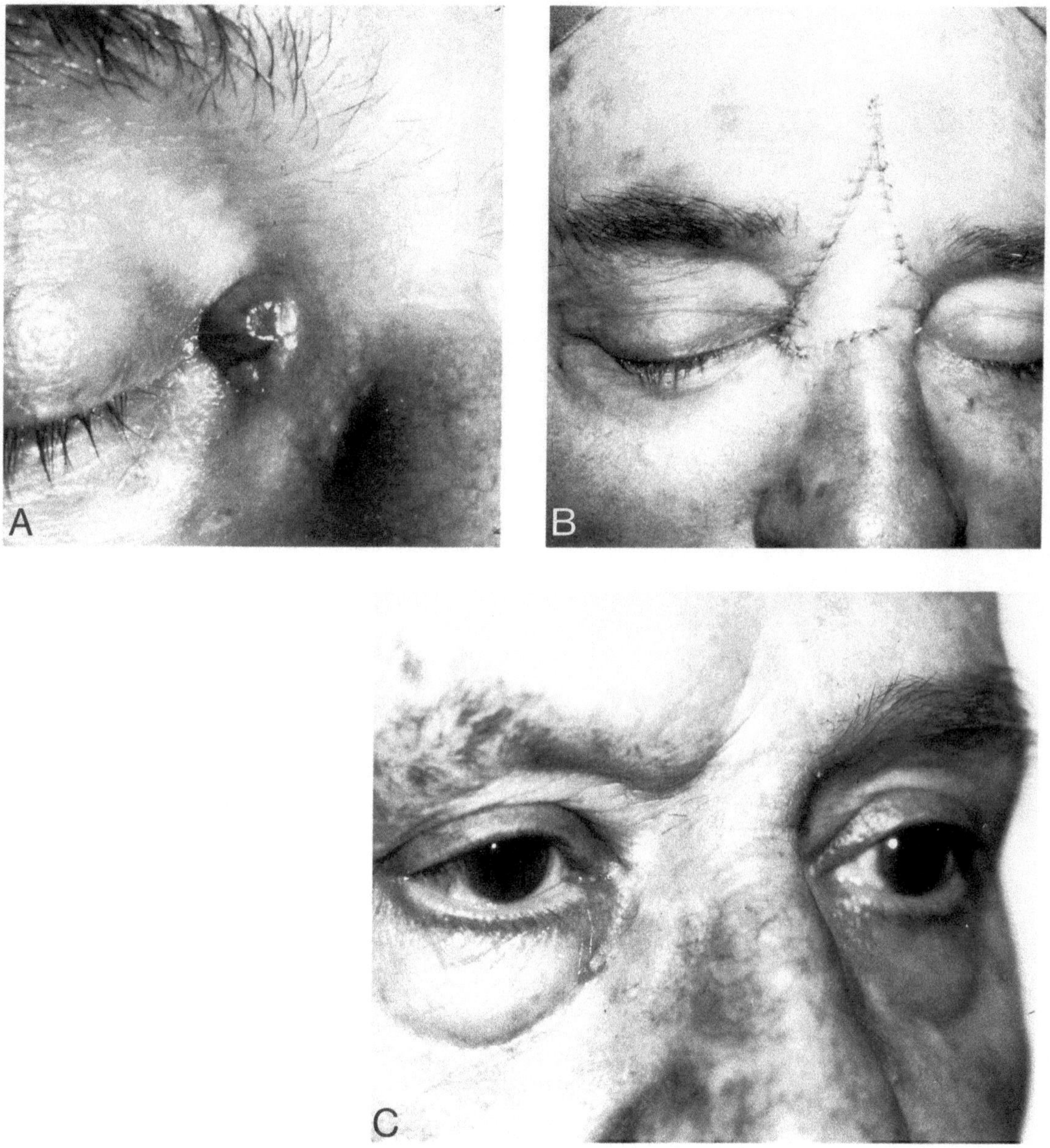

Fig. 4.34 A–C. Medial canthus – Mustardé V-Y advancement flap. **A** Papulo-pearly BCC in a 63-year-old man. **B** The glabellar flap is advanced without difficulty into the medial canthal area, where its tip should be thinned. **C** At 2 years

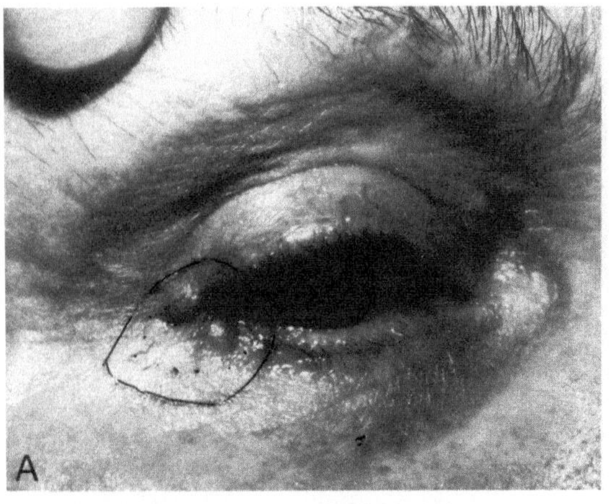

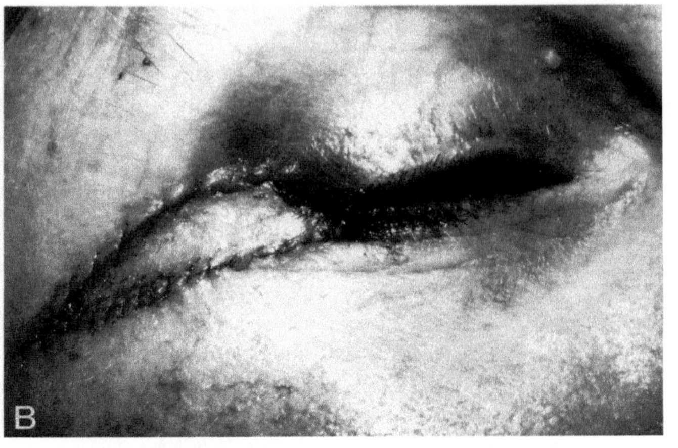

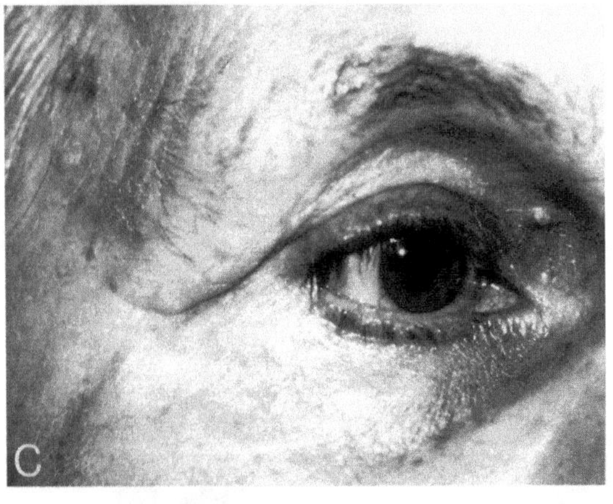

Fig. 4.35 A–C. Lateral canthus – kite flap. **A** A sclerosing BCC invading the palpebral commissure in a 64-year-old woman. **B** A kite flap is combined with a flap of conjunctiva to repair the defect. **C** At 6 months there is minimal deformity

The Forehead and Eyebrows

Forehead skin is homogeneous and elastic, and scars in this area are usually of good quality and are easily hidden in the local wrinkles. The arrangement of horizontal wrinkles should be carefully preserved. Eyebrow reconstruction must take into account the oblique direction of growth of the individual hairs. The symmetry of the two brows must be carefully respected.

Elliptical excision is only rarely indicated. A horizontal resection creates a significant risk of permanently elevating the adjacent eyebrow. However, elliptical excision is possible for small lesions when skin excess is present, provided the lesion is located in the upper half of the forehead (Fig. 4.36). To be effective undermining must be carried out between the skin and the frontal muscle to which it is adherent. A vertically oriented ellipse may result in a distinctly visible scar.

The H-flap is the technique of choice for the repair of small and moderately sized defects of the forehead. The incisions for the advancement flaps are placed in wrinkle lines or along the borders of the eyebrows. There is usually some pleating upon closure due to the unequal lengths of the margins, but this resolves rapidly and the results are generally excellent (Fig. 4.37 and Color Plate IA, p. 108). The forehead skin is remarkably elastic and allows the repair of large defects.

Near the scalp a T-design is useful since the vertical limit can be extended into the hair-bearing area (Fig. 4.38). In the area of the lateral forehead the H-flap is very useful to prevent vertical displacement of the hairline and eyebrow. A triangle can be excised from the area of the crow's-feet to facilitate adjustment of the skin margins (Fig. 4.39).

The full-thickness skin graft may be indicated for defects that are too extensive for local flaps. The frontal muscle should be preserved to allow wrinkles to form in the graft. If the muscle must be sacrificed the graft will be made more visible by its immobility (Fig. 4.40).

The eyebrows deserve special comment. Care must be taken to avoid interruption of their continuity and creation of distortion, but a slight reduction in the length of the eyebrow will not be noticeable.

The technique of choice to repair the eyebrow following excision of a BCC is the H-flap (Fig. 5.3, p. 88). The incisions that cross the eyebrow are directed obliquely, parallel to the follicles, to avoid damaging these structures. The flaps are undercut in a plane deep to the follicles.

When the lesion extends above the eyebrow and/or is too wide for an H-flap, a kite flap can be taken from the forehead if there is good transverse laxity. Dissection must be precise to preserve the frontal branch of the facial nerve and keep a sufficient blood supply to the skin island through the underlying muscle (Fig. 4.41).

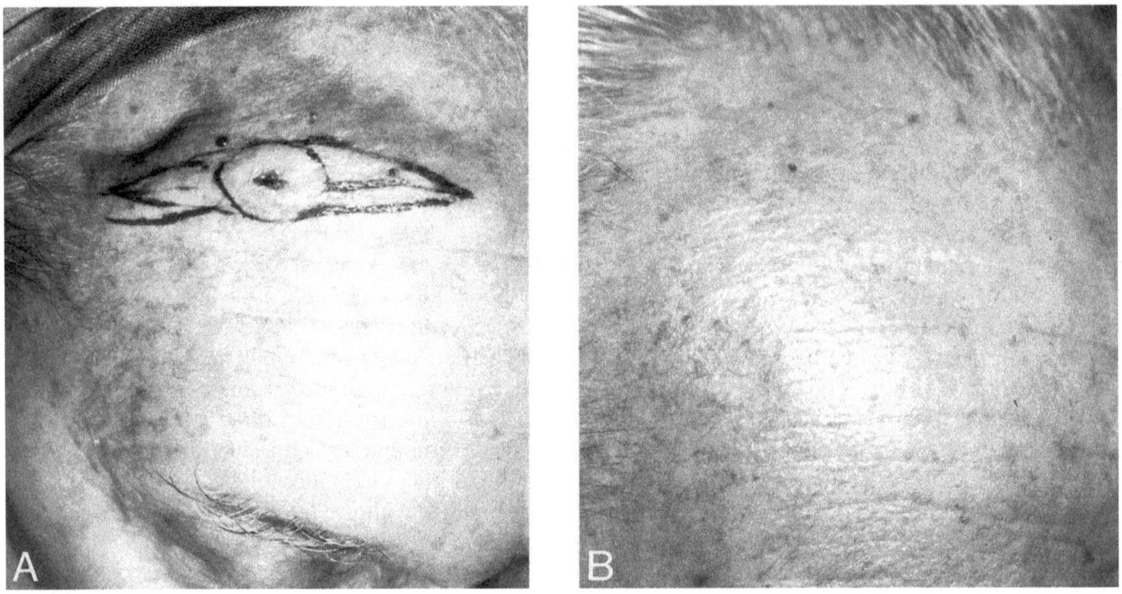

Fig. 4.36. Upper forehead – elliptical excision. In this 78-year-old man an elliptical excision carefully placed in the skin wrinkles has produced an invisible repair

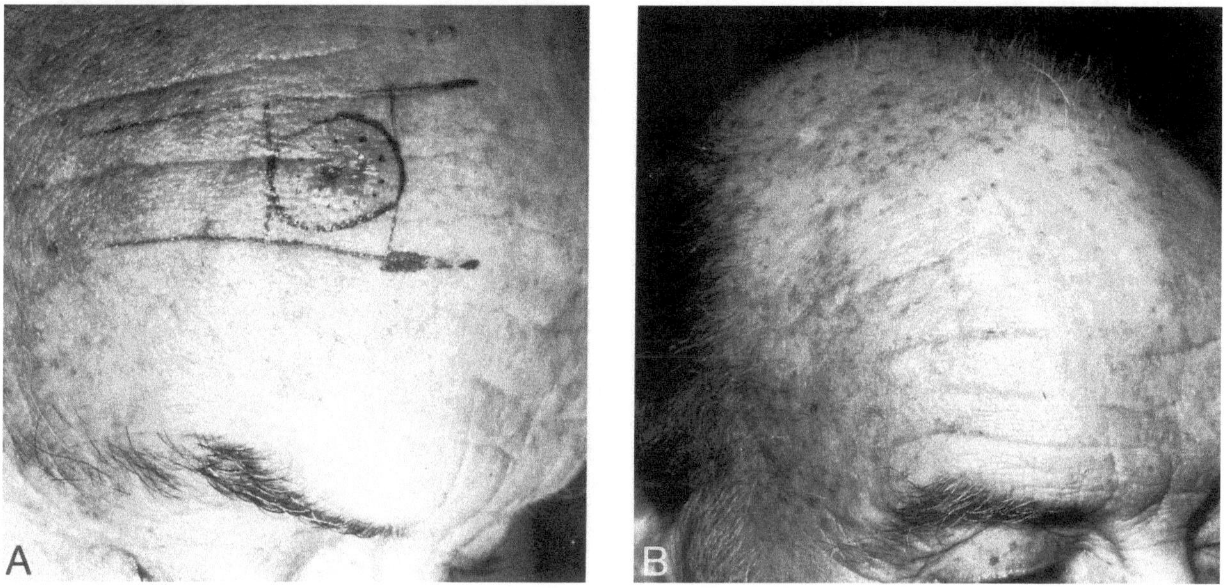

Fig. 4.37 A, B. Forehead – H-flap. **A** In a 77-year-old man, a BCC of 6 months standing. The horizontal incisions must be placed in existing wrinkles when these are well defined, even if this extends the size of the excision. **B** At 3 months the appearance is already acceptable

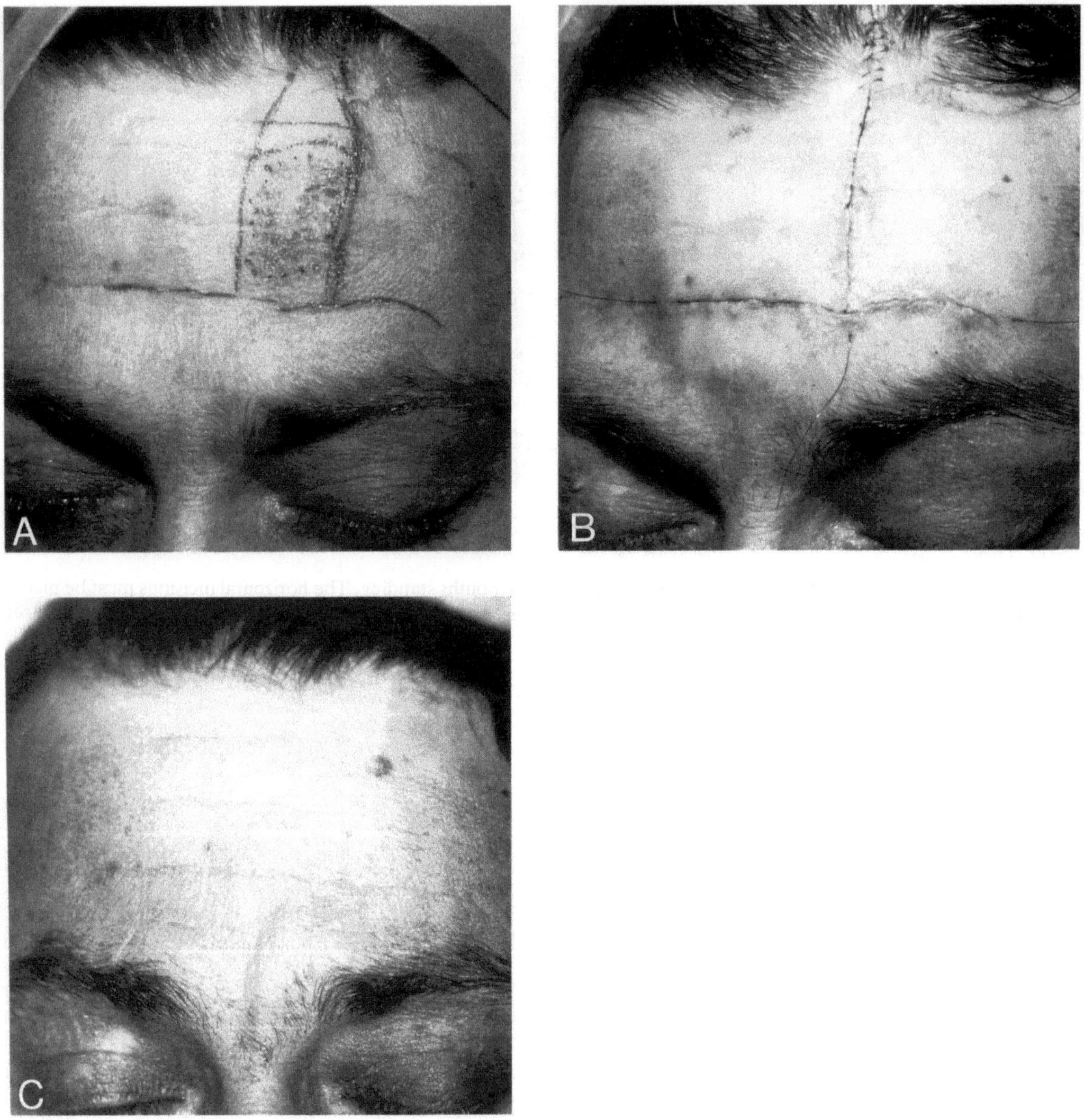

Fig. 4.38 A–C. Forehead – T-plasty. **A** A multifocal BCC in a 34-year-old man treated for 4 years by cryotherapy: because the lesion is situated near the hairline the vertical incision can be extended into the scalp. **B** Following wide undermining, advancement, and closure in two layers with a running subcuticular, suture for the skin. **C** At 3 years

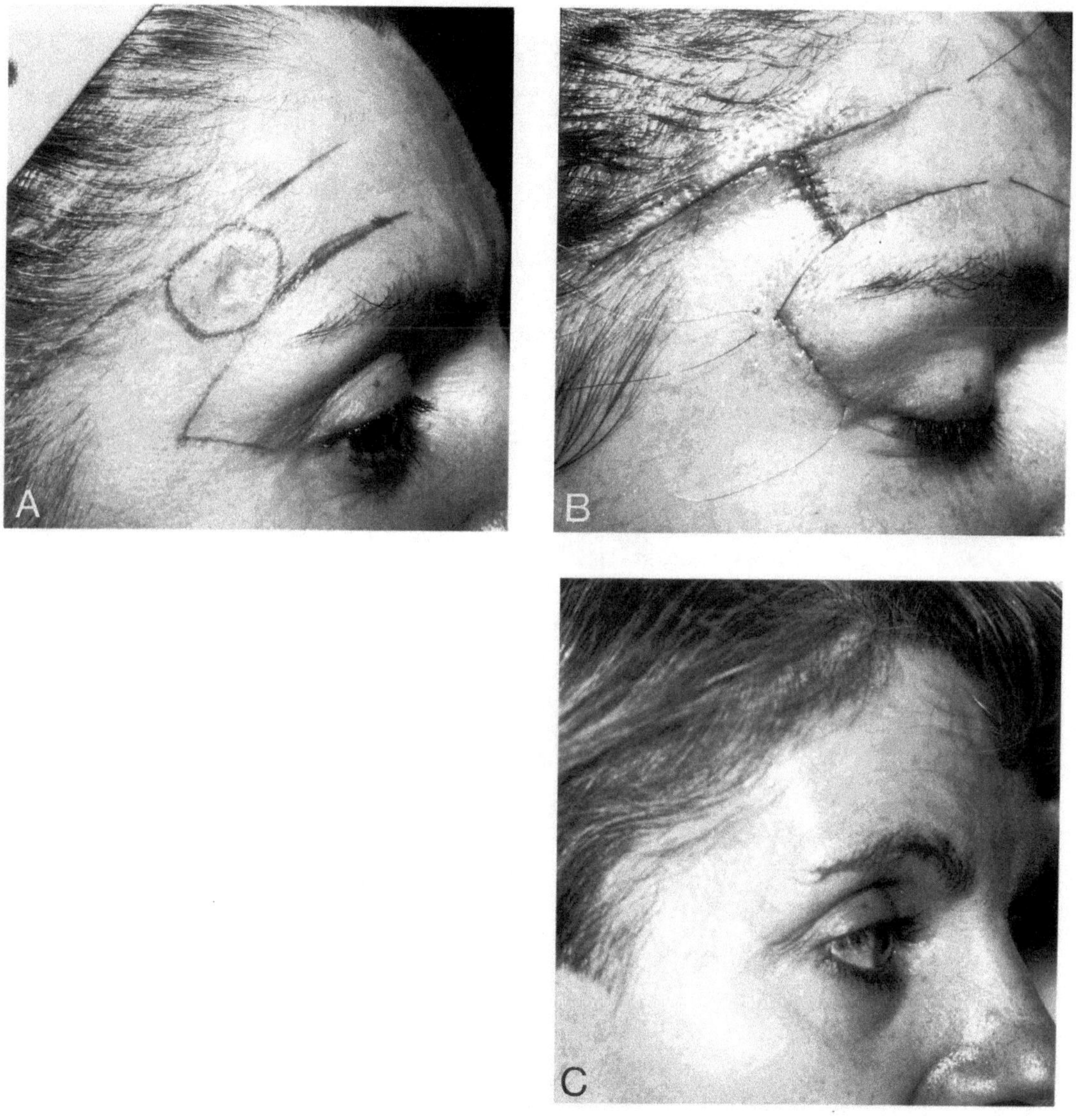

Fig. 4.39 A–C. Lateral forehead – H-flap. **A** A 48-year-old patient with a BCC situated between the hairline and the lateral eyebrow, which must not be displaced. **B** The H-flap provides a good repair with placement of the dog-ear in the crow's-feet area. **C** At 2 years the result is judged "excellent"

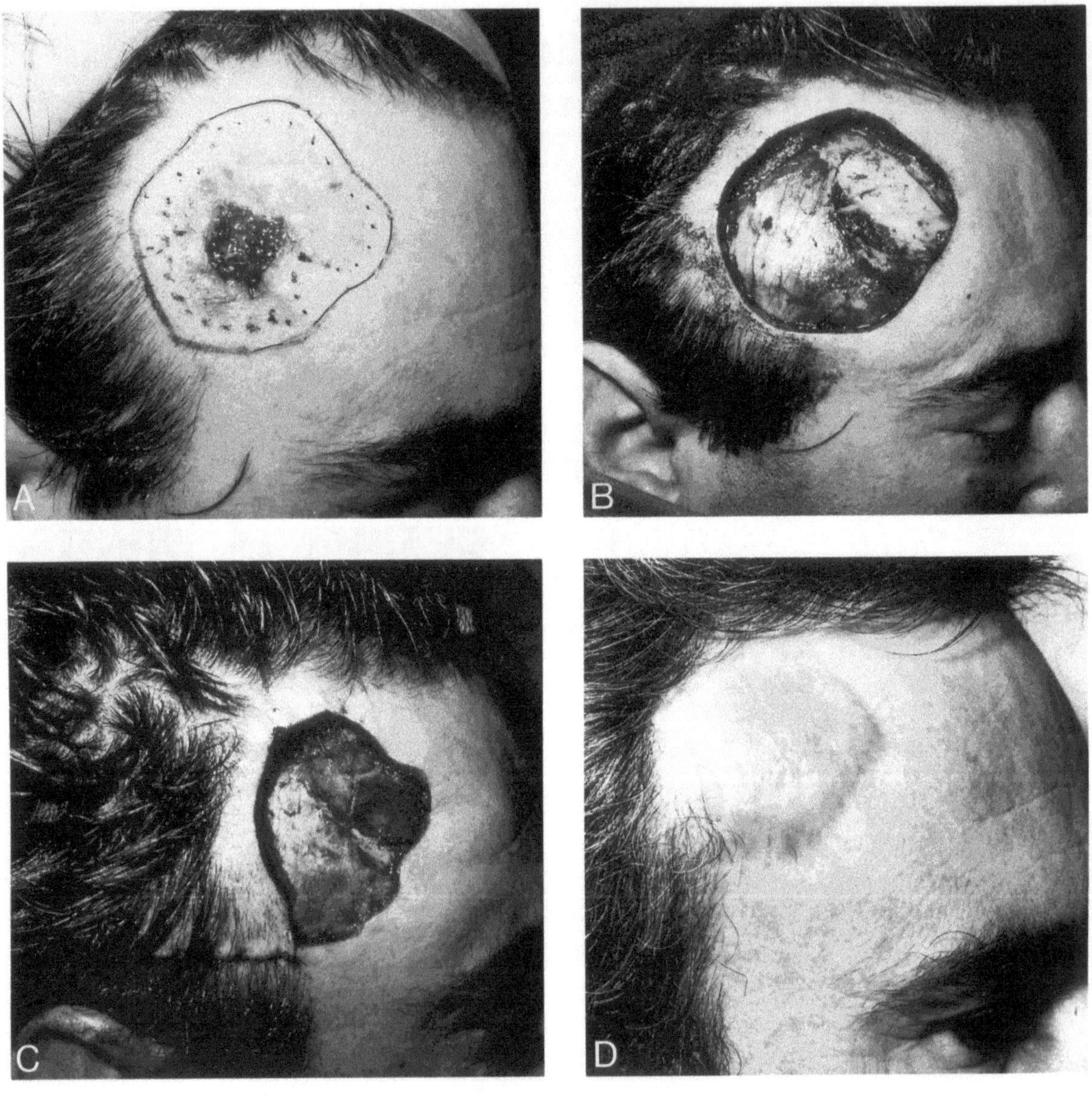

Fig. 4.40 A–D. Forehead – full-thickness skin graft. **A** This 43-year-old patient presented with a vast, ulcerated BCC that developed at the site of a traumatic lesion. **B** The excision exposes temporal muscle and frontal bone. **C** A posterior scalp rotation flap reestablishes the hairline. A temporal muscle flap covers the exposed bone and is in turn resurfaced with a retroauricular full-thickness graft. **D** At 9 months the graft is very visible, but the appearance should improve with time

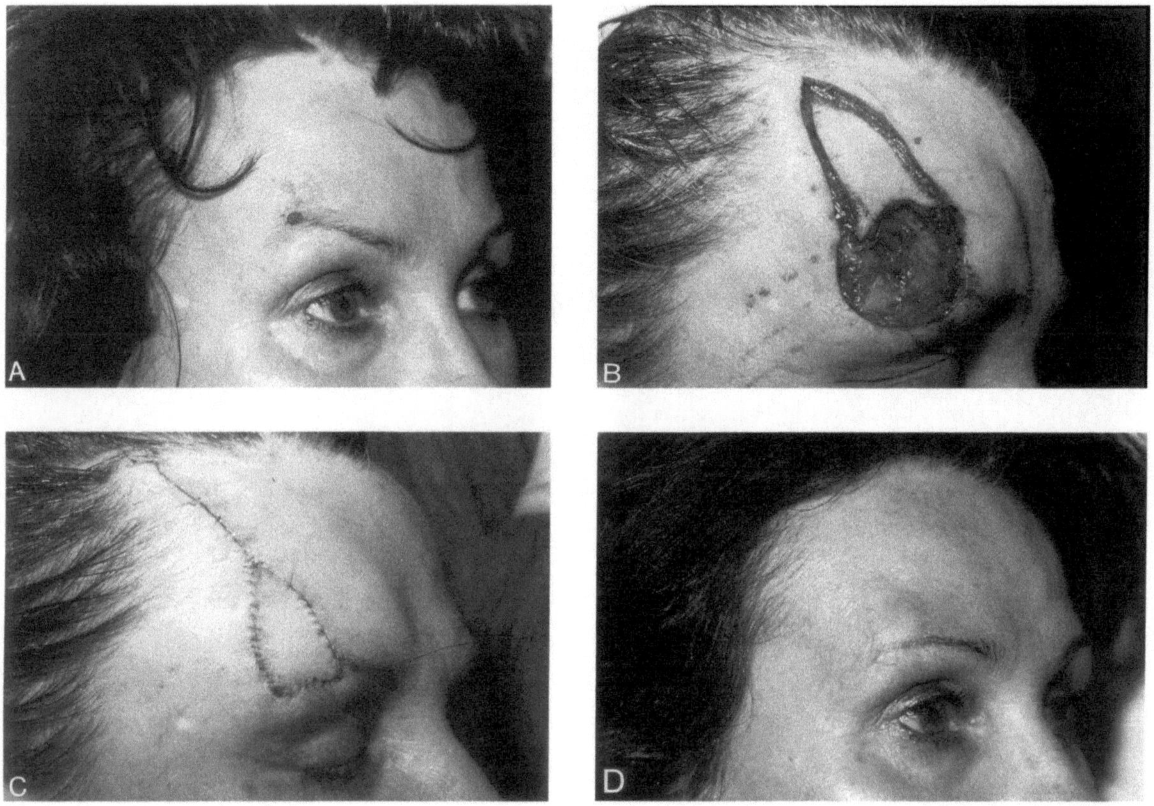

Fig. 4.41. A Patient aged 52, presenting with a basocell carcinoma of the eyebrow. This lesion has recurred after two previous surgical excision, five years and seven years ago. **B** A wide excision was carried out. Since some laxity was present above it, a kite-flap based on the frontalis muscle was elevated. **C** After adjustement of the kite-flap. **D** One year after excision and repair

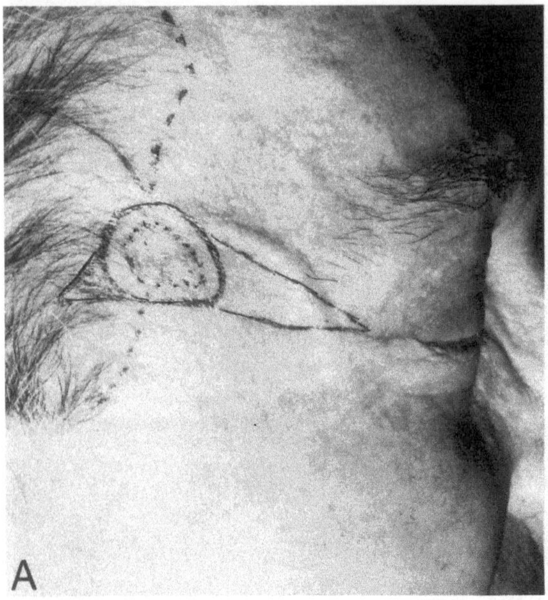

Fig. 4.42 A, B. Temporal area – elliptical excision. **A** A recurrent BCC, 2 years following electrodesiccation in a 65-year-old man. **B** The skin laxity in the temporal area allows use of an ellipse oriented in the direction of the crow's-feet. The hairline must be carefully aligned

The Temporal Region

The skin is usually lax in this area and marked by well-defined wrinkles or crow's-feet.

An elliptical excision often yields very good results when it is correctly oriented. Undermining must be wide and care must be taken to avoid injury to the frontal branch of the facial nerve. This branch lies in contact with the muscular layer and ascends to a point just above the lateral end of the eyebrow (Fig. 4.42).

The LLL-flap provides a good alternative when the skin cannot be closed primarily, but nearer to the forehead the H-flap is a better solution (Fig. 4.39).

The rotation flap is very useful when the defect borders on the temporal scalp. A long curving incision hidden in the hair-bearing skin will provide the necessary cover (Figs. 4.43 and 4.44).

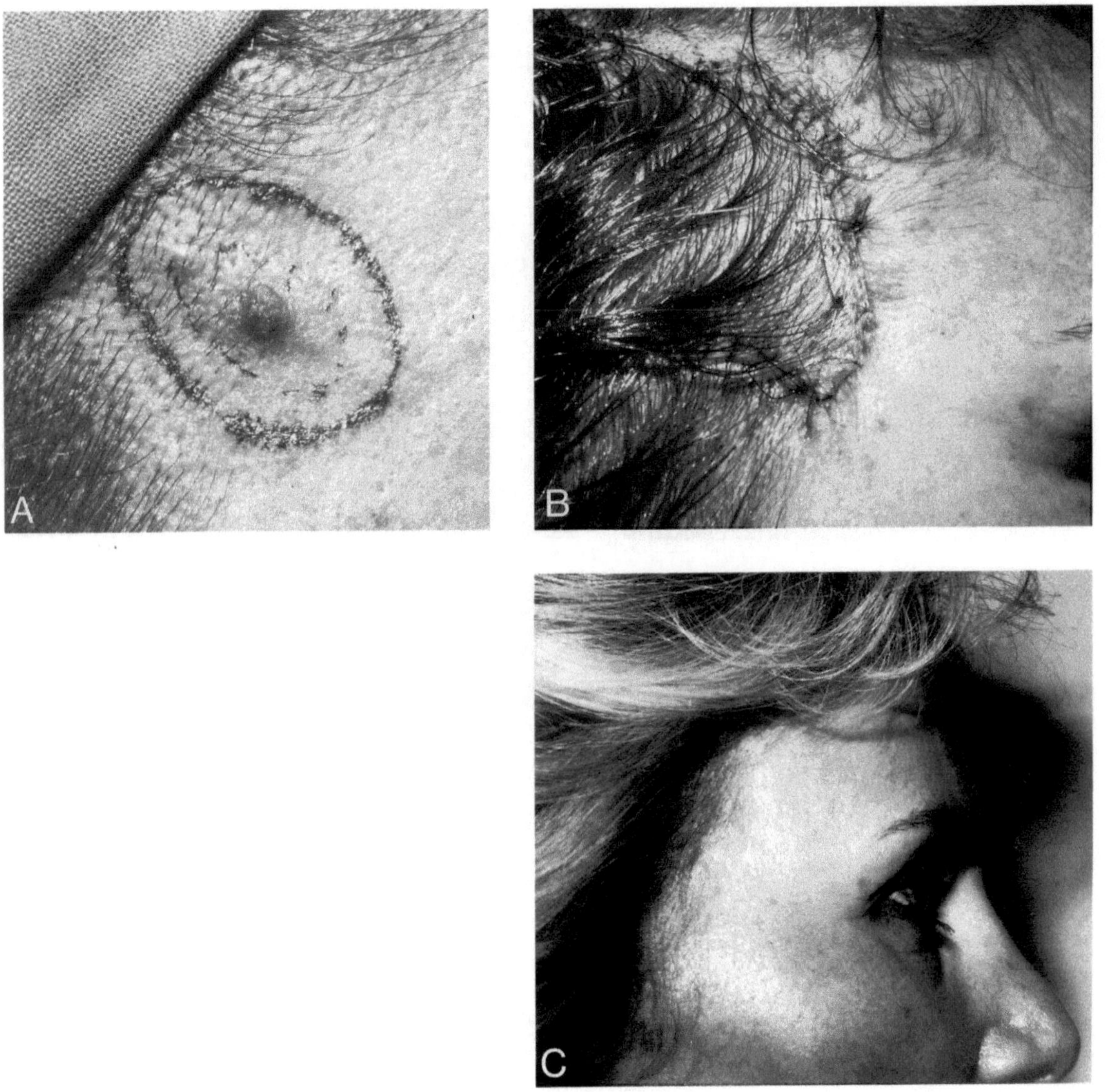

Fig. 4.43 A–C. Temporal area – rotation flap. **A** A 47-year-old woman with a BCC near the hairline. **B** A large rotation flap has reestablished the hairline. **C** At 4 years the hairline is normal and the scar is scarcely visible. The aesthetic result is judged "excellent"

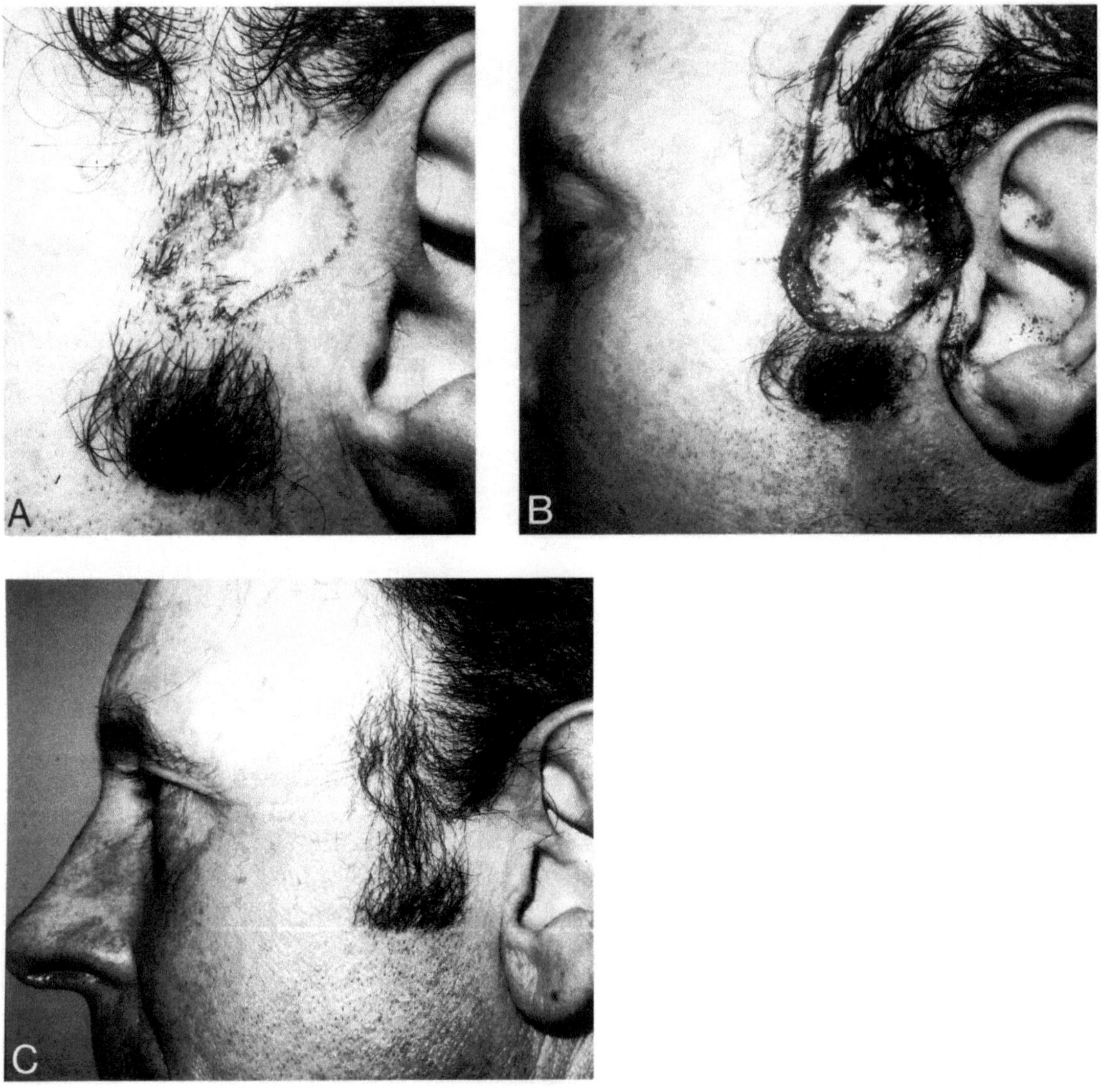

Fig. 4.44 A–C. Temporal area – rotation flap. **A** A large plaque of ulcerated BCC recurring 4 years following electrodesiccation in a 53-year-old man. **B** A scalp rotation flap is raised above the defect. **C** At 3 years there is no alopecia and the scar is not visible

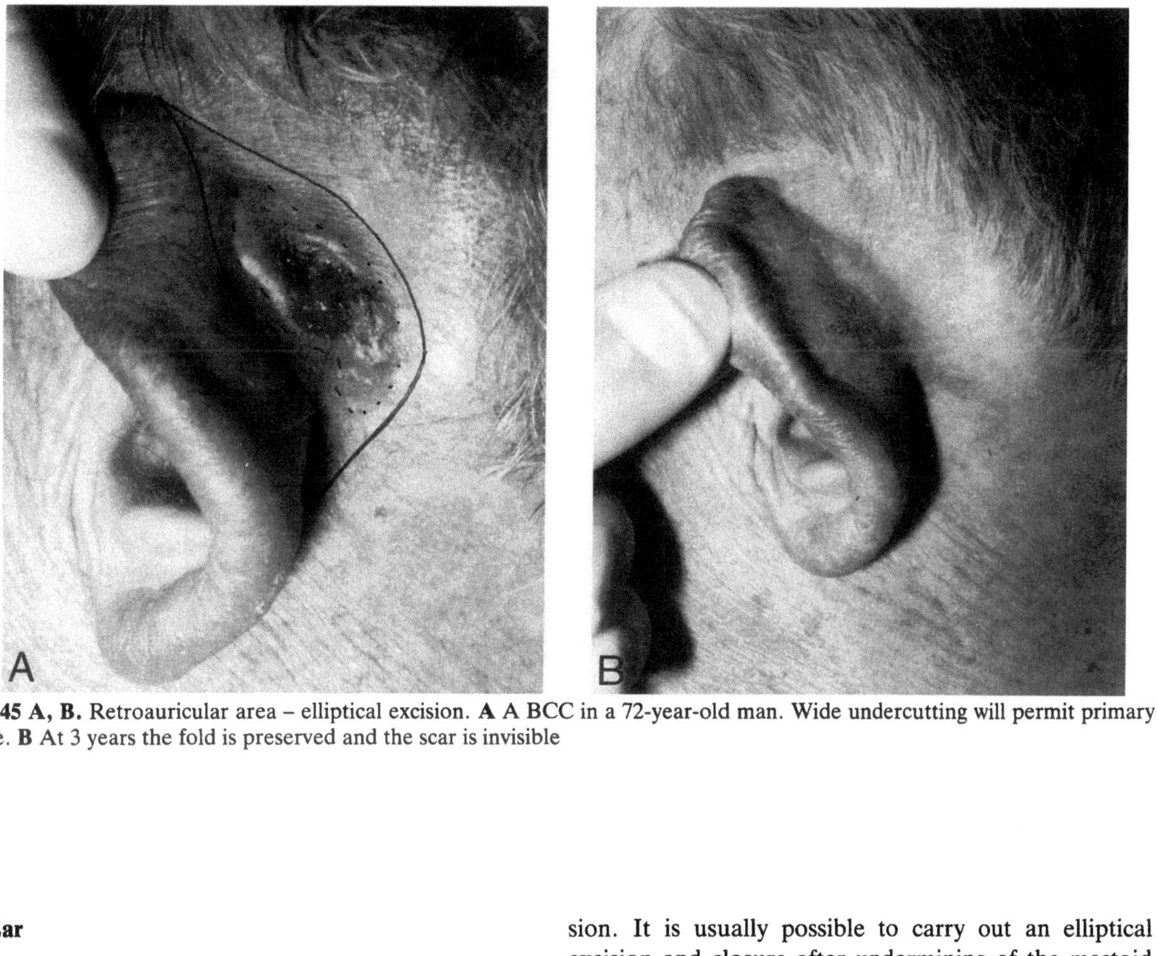

Fig. 4.45 A, B. Retroauricular area – elliptical excision. **A** A BCC in a 72-year-old man. Wide undercutting will permit primary closure. **B** At 3 years the fold is preserved and the scar is invisible

The Ear

Squamous cell carcinoma is more frequent than BCC at this location but the problem is essentially the same: to carry out an adequate excision without destroying the complex architecture of the ear.

The anterior skin is strongly adherent to the cartilage, which often must be removed as well. Repair may be carried out with a full-thickness skin graft applied to the deep surface of the posterior skin or with a flap raised from the retroauricular fold and transposed anteriorly through a transfixing incision.

The posterior skin is more easily separated from the cartilage, which can often be preserved during the excision. It is usually possible to carry out an elliptical excision and closure after undermining of the mastoid and retroauricular skin (Fig. 4.45).

Lesions of the *helical rim* are the most frequent due to actinic exposure. Even slight irregularity in this area is highly visible. A preferred technique consists of a full-thickness wedge excision (Fig. 4.46), which produces a normal ear of somewhat smaller size. Asymmetry of the ears goes unnoticed.

When the resection exceeds one quarter of the helix, other possibilities for reconstruction include a contralateral auricular cartilage graft covered by a retroauricular flap, or a composite ear graft, which has the advantage of creating two symmetrical, but smaller ears.

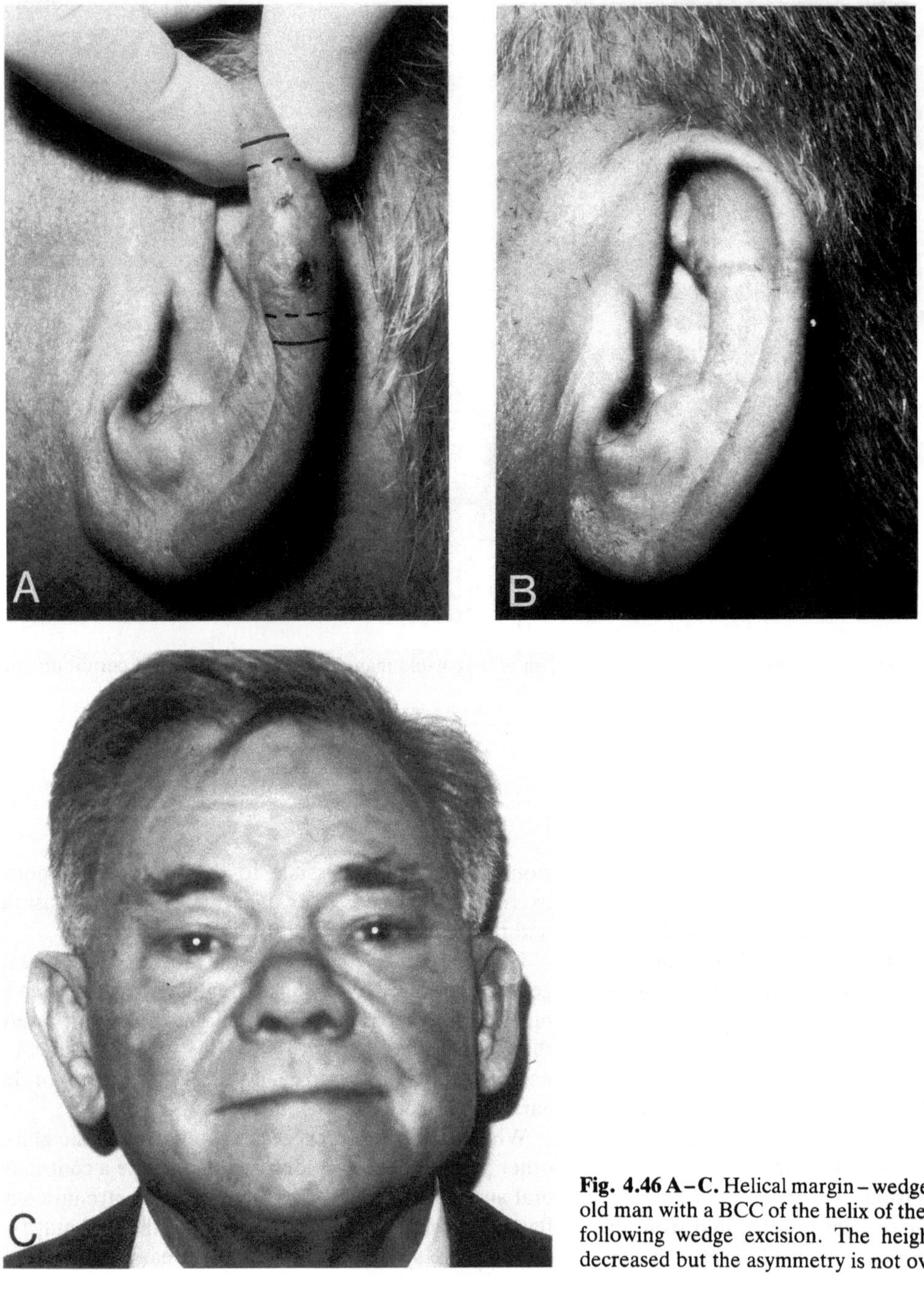

Fig. 4.46 A–C. Helical margin – wedge resection. **A** A 75-year-old man with a BCC of the helix of the ear. **B** and **C** Two years following wedge excision. The height of the ear has been decreased but the asymmetry is not overly conspicuous

Deep Tumor Extension

Malignant infiltration of deep tissues can have catastrophic consequences. In these situations even bone provides only a temporary barrier. Dangerous areas are those where infiltrating tumor can reach the brain and other vital structures. These include:

1. The auricular and parotid areas where the internal ear and facial nerve may be affected
2. The nasal and orbital regions where tumor may invade the orbital fat and ethmoid sinus and eventually the base of the skull
3. The forehead region, particularly vulnerable because the bone is just beneath the skin and because the rapidly adherent lesion often seems noninvasive (Binstock et al. 1981)

Resection must be wide in these areas and should extend past the plane of invasion. Appreciation of the deep margin is often difficult, especially since bony invasion is poorly demonstrated on roentgenograms. On several occasions we have discovered a completely perforated frontal bone with invasion of the dura mater when the radiographs had suggested only minimal bony involvement.

Clinically fixed lesions necessitate deep resections, especially in the frontal region where neurosurgical support must be available if it becomes necessary to sacrifice full-thickness bone and dura mater (Fig. 4.47). If indicated, it is possible to resect subjacent cerebral tissue or the longitudinal sinus in its anterior portion. The dura mater is repaired with a patch of cranial periosteum or lyophilized dura. Frontal bone is reconstructed with a split rib graft (Fig. 4.48), a split cranial bone, or, in certain cases, with a methyl methacrylate prosthesis.

Recurrences are catastrophic and necessitate radical excision.

The Concept of Aesthetic Units

The face can be considered to be composed of anatomic or aesthetic units which should be respected in such procedures as skin grafts. According to this concept, the complete aesthetic unit should be resurfaced when any significant portion requires reconstruction. For example, one would graft the whole upper lip or eyelid when a defect involves half the surface area. This concept is valid only in very particular circumstances such as in treating facial burns. In fact, one should carefully choose the simplest repair that will restore harmony, even if only half the unit is treated. The patient shown in Fig. 4.31 demonstrates that a partial graft of the lower eyelid may be perfectly integrated into the remaining lid.

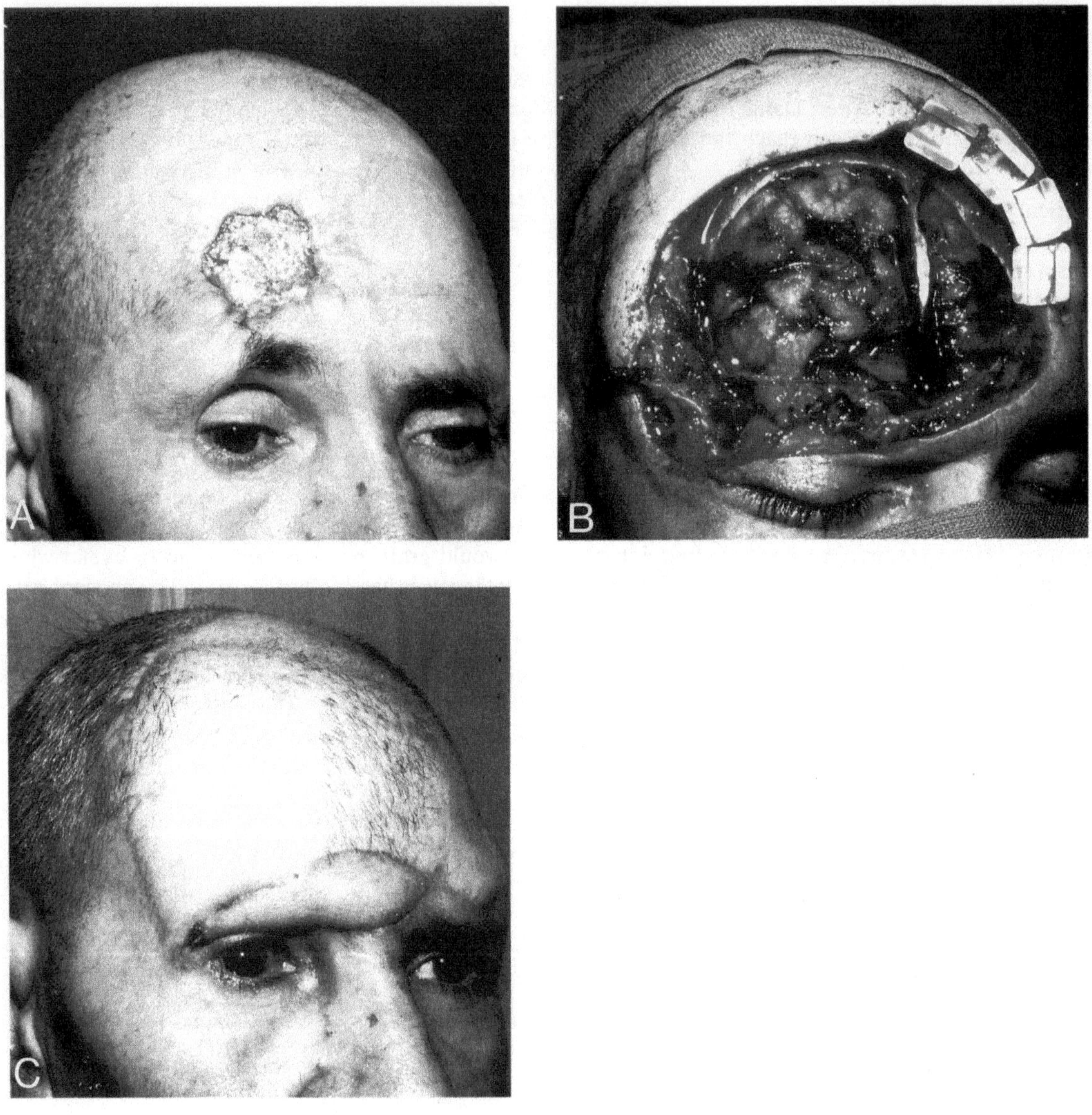

Fig. 4.47 A–C. Invasive forehead lesion. **A** A 60-year-old patient presenting with an ulcerated lesion of the forehead of several years standing. There is bone invasion. **B** After en bloc resection of skin and frontal bone, the dura mater is noted to be involved with tumor and is excised. **C** The dura mater has been reconstructed with a graft of cranial periosteum, the skull defect with a methyl methacrylate implant, and cover has been provided by a large scalp flap. Appearance at 3 months

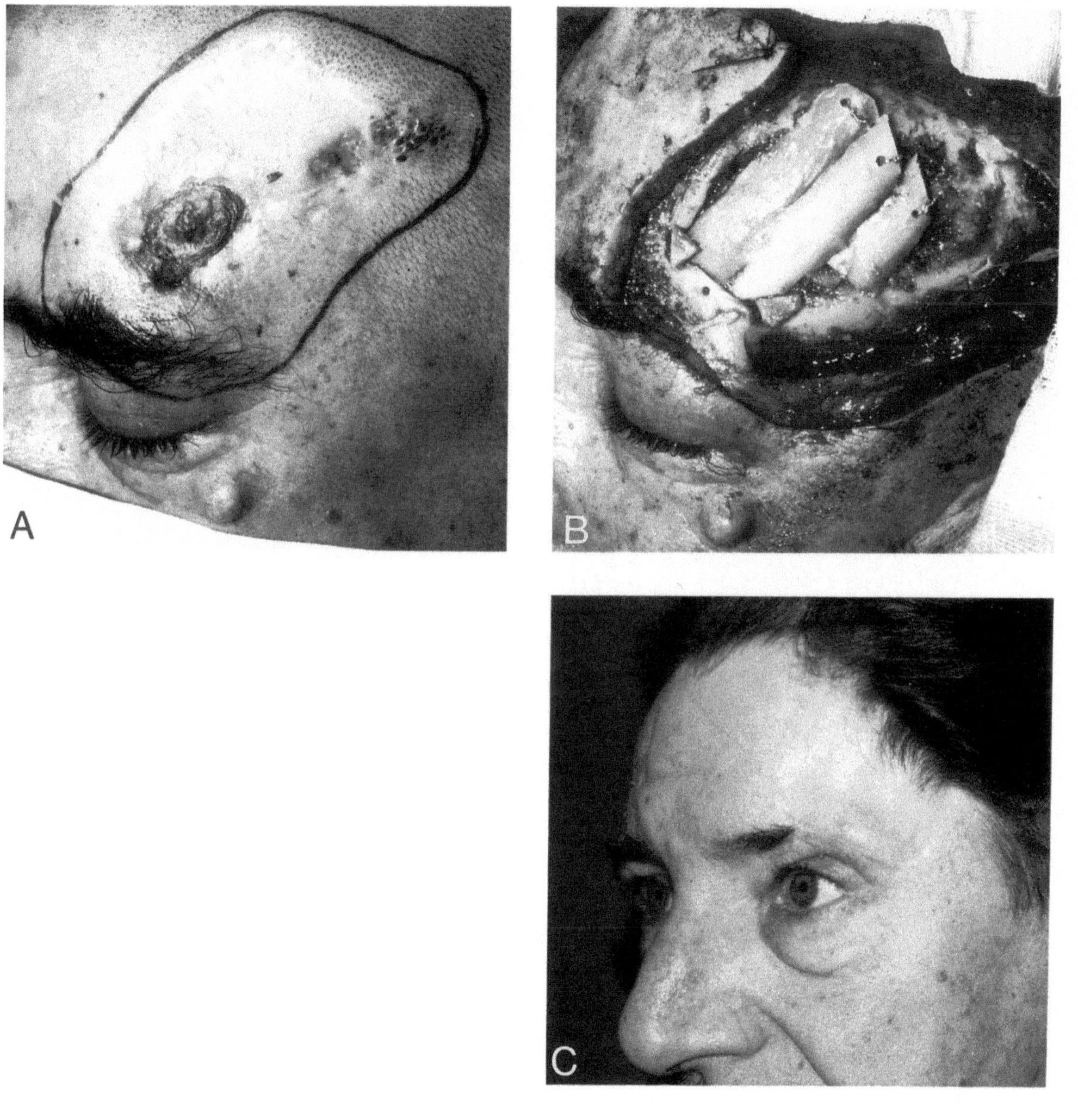

Fig. 4.48 A–C. Invasive forehead lesion. **A** A 52-year-old man with a BCC that has recurred following grafting and radiotheraphy. **B** Following frontal resection, the bone reconstruction is carried out with rib grafts and cover is provided by a scalping forehead flap. **C** At 5 years the principal deformity is the loss of half the eyebrow. An hair-bearing strip graft was refused by the patient

Chapter 5 **Analysis of a Series of 225 Cases**

This analysis is based on a series of 225 BCCs of the face with a minimum of 3 years' follow-up. This interval was considered appropriate as the majority of recurrences appear by the 2nd year (Taylor and Barisoni 1973).

The series includes 210 patients operated on between 1969 and 1981. One hundred nine additional patients operated on during this period and accounting for 127 lesions were excluded because they did not meet the conditions for follow-up. From 1981 to 1987 a further 298 patients were treated, some of whom appear in the illustrations, but they were not included in the present series.

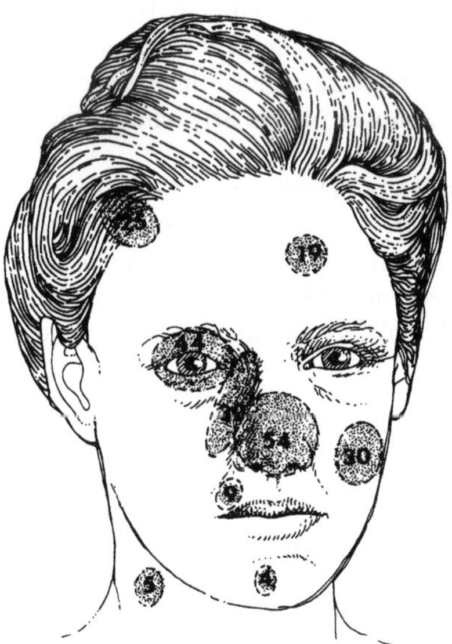

Fig. 5.1. The lesions in the present series are located predominantly at the center of the face

All patients were operated on by the author according to techniques described in Chaps. 2 and 3. *The great majority were treated on an outpatient basis.*

Admission was indicated on 17 occasions for patients who were especially fearful or fragile or who had extensive lesions. In these cases local anesthesia was preceded by a premedication and facilitated by brief general anesthesia using propanidid (Epontol, Théraplix Laboratories) during infiltration. Propanidid is not a respiratory depressant and does not necessitate intubation. Administrated intravenously, it produces a brief loss of consciousness which the patient often does not remember. This light anesthesia is well tolerated, especially by the elderly. Three of these 17 patients were discharged on the same day, wide awake and accompanied by family or friends, ten were discharged 24 h post-op, and four patients were kept for 5 days until removal of the sutures.

Lesions and Types of Repair

The lesions encountered and the types of repair employed were in accordance with the data presented in other publications (Burg et al. 1975; Chernosky 1978; Hayes 1972; Jackson 1973; Porte et al. 1979; Sakura and Calamel 1979; Taylor and Barisoni 1973; Zeller and Touraine 1982) in terms of size, location, type, and classification into primary vs. recurrent lesions.

The tumor localization was mainly centrofacial, as illustrated by Fig. 5.1, involving the nose, the eyelids, the nasolabial folds, and the forehead.

The lesions were usually greater than 3 mm in diameter (91.2%) and often exceeded 10 mm (43.6%), with lesions smaller than 3 mm accounting for only 8.9% of cases. Obviously, the surgical defects were correspondingly larger to allow for adequate margins.

In this series of 225 BCCs the majority were nodular and ulcerative, but we also observed 31 sclerosing and 11 multicentric lesions.

There were 34 recurrent lesions (19.1%) which had been subjected to various types of initial treatment: to surgery (3), to electrocoagulation or liquid nitrogen (17), to radiotherapy (14), and occasionally to combinations of these. We observed five tumors that appeared following irradiation of hemangiomas in childhood; three of these were extensive (see Fig. 4.4), and one led to an enucleation in a young woman. There were no instances of metastasis in our series.

The surgical techniques employed are listed in Table 5.1, from which it is evident that the use of local tissue predominated.

Table 5.1. Techniques of repair used in 225 cases

Technique	No. of cases	%
Elliptical excision with undermining	65	28.9
Local flap	129	57.3
Distant flap	5	2.2
Full-thickness skin graft	26	11.6

Oncologic Results

In 225 BCCs with a minimum of 3 years' follow-up we had five recurrences (2.22%). These lesions were dispersed, as shown in Fig. 5.2, and specific conclusions cannot be drawn.

Recurrent lesions have a bad reputation [15% recurrence following re-excision as reported by Rank and Wakefield (1959) and 24% for Hayes (1972)], as do poorly delimited tumors such as the sclerosing BCC. We noted two recurrences among the 34 sclerosing BCCs, and it is interesting that among the 34 recurrent lesions only two reappeared following excision (Elton 1975; Epstein 1974).

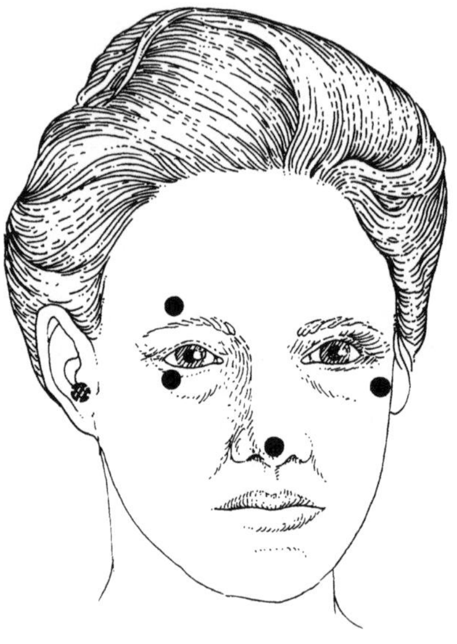

Fig. 5.2. Location of the five tumors that recurred

Areas such as the nasolabial fold and the medial canthus are considered especially subject to recurrence. We did not observe a single recurrence in these cases, perhaps because excision was particularly wide in these problem areas (see Fig. 4.5).

We agree with Pascal et al. (1968) that *the only serious risk factor is an inadequate excision.* The factors just cited above serve simply increase the probability of an insufficiently extensive resection. The technical details concerning excision and histologic examination are found on pages 7–11.

Aesthetic Results

The quality of the aesthetic results or, if one prefers, the evaluation of the sequelae of the surgical treatment, is very important in the comparison of results with those of other series. Such an aesthetic assessment appears justified in the treatment of facial lesions that are cured in 98% of cases. It goes without saying that *oncologic risks should not be taken to improve the aesthetic results.*

However, appropriate cancer treatment does not exclude an effort to minimize the aesthetic sequelae.

It is curious that no attempt was made to assess the aesthetic results of the treatment of malignant skin tumors prior to our first publication on this subject in 1980 (Marchac and Duport), with the exception of a brief evaluation of eight cases by Epstein (1974). Such assessments are complicated by the fact that a good result may not be considered as such by a second observer.

In an attempt to establish a certain objectivity, we judge our results in the following manner: the patient is placed at a distance of approximately 50 cm from the observer, or common conversational distance, under good daylight illumination. The evaluation is made not by the surgeon, who will tend to take into account the difficulty of the repair, but by a neutral observer who has no knowledge of the preoperative condition or the techniques used for repair.

The existence of deformity, asymmetry, visible scars, or a change in skin texture or color forms the basis for classification of the results according to the following scale:

- *Excellent*: absence of deformity, asymmetry, or visible scar. There is no visible evidence of surgery. Excellent results are illustrated in Figs. 5.3 and 4.29.
- *Good*: there is visible evidence of surgery, such as deformity, asymmetry, or a visible scar. However, this is minimal and inconspicuous. The scar is inconspicuous in the patient shown in Fig. 4.9, but there is also a slight deformity. The scar is more visible in Fig. 4.5, while the patient in Fig. 5.4 has asymmetry of the two lower eyelids.
- *Mediocre*: the repair is clearly visible and one promptly notes the abnormality. The patient in Fig. 5.5 has undergone full-thickness grafting of the nose, which has a patchwork appearance, and the flap in Fig. 5.6 is clearly visible. The lip of the patient in Fig. 5.7 is distinctly asymmetric.
- *Poor*: the aesthetic result is obviously displeasing, with the repair very visible. The patient in Fig. 5.8 was judged to have a poor result. We do not consider this a failure, as it was perhaps the best possible result under the circumstances. However, from a purely aesthetic perspective the result is poor.

Table 5.2. Aesthetic results in 225 cases

Result	No. of cases	%	
Excellent	144	64	93
Good	66	29	
Mediocre	13	6	
Poor	2	1	

These criteria were applied to the 225 lesions comprising the series and the evaluations were made by a number of plastic surgeons who were seeing the patients for the first time. Satisfactory results, including excellent and good outcomes, represent 93% of the total (see Table 2).

It is interesting to analyze in detail the 15 unsatisfactory results, in which the following techniques were employed:

- Elliptical excision – 5%
- Local flap – 15%
- Distant flap – 50%
- Skin graft – 30%

Elliptical excision led to only one mediocre result, a resection in an upper lip resulting in a vertical scar and asymmetry, similar to that shown in Fig. 5.7.

Local flaps rarely yield unsatisfactory results but, as expected, distant flaps used to close vast defects often produce poor aesthetic results.

In contrast, full-thickness skin grafts are widely considered to provide satisfactory results, yet despite 100% take they were associated with unsatisfactory results in 20% of the cases in which they were used. These were due in part to depressions secondary to the nonreplacement of lost subcutaneous tissue and in part to differences in color or texture.

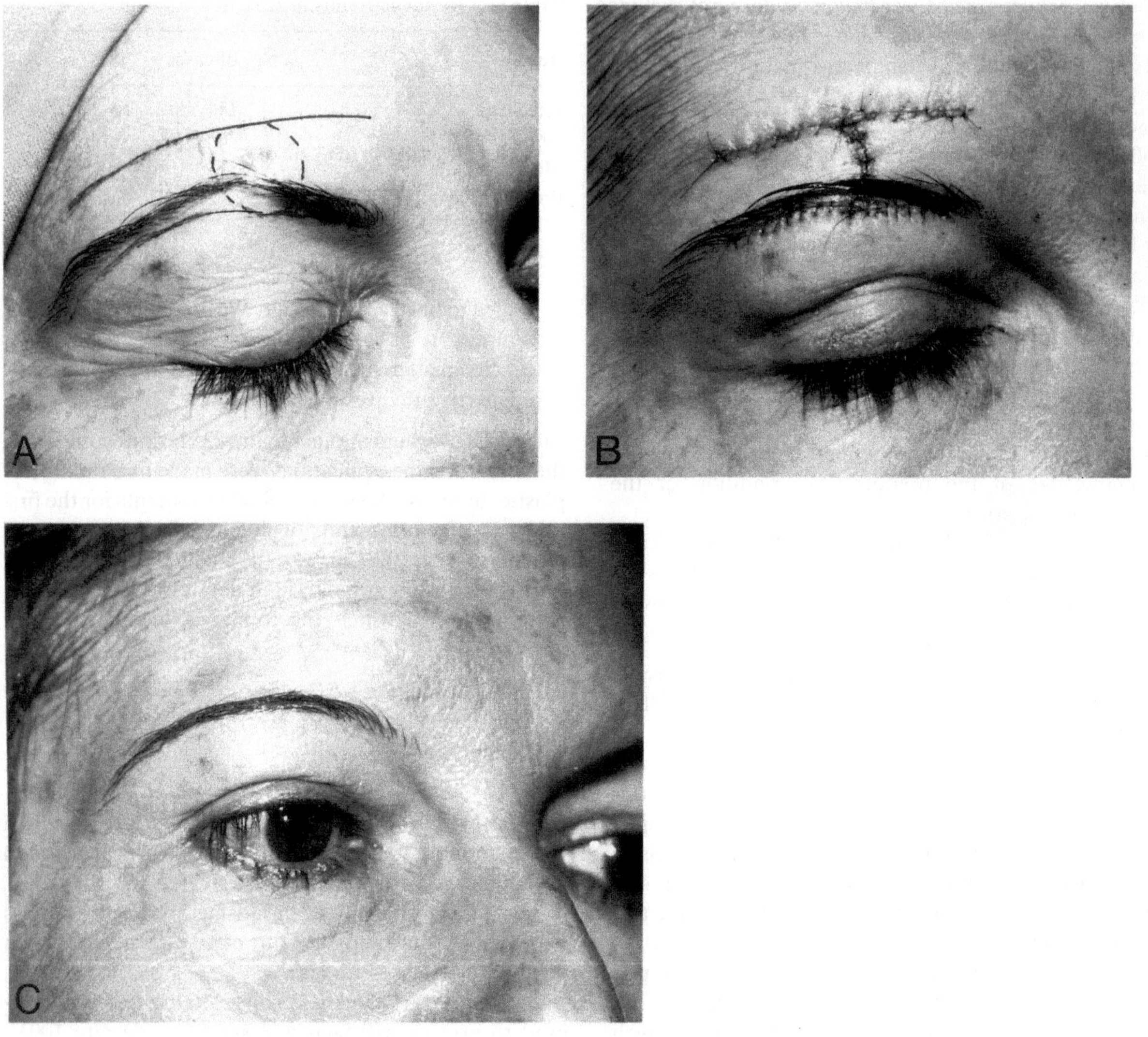

Fig. 5.3 A–C. An "excellent" aesthetic result. **A** A 48-year-old patient presenting with a BCC of the forehead that involves the eyebrow. An H-flap is designed. **B** The H-flap has allowed reconstruction of the brow. **C** Four years later the patient considers herself "mutilated" despite the symmetry, mobility, and satisfactory appearance

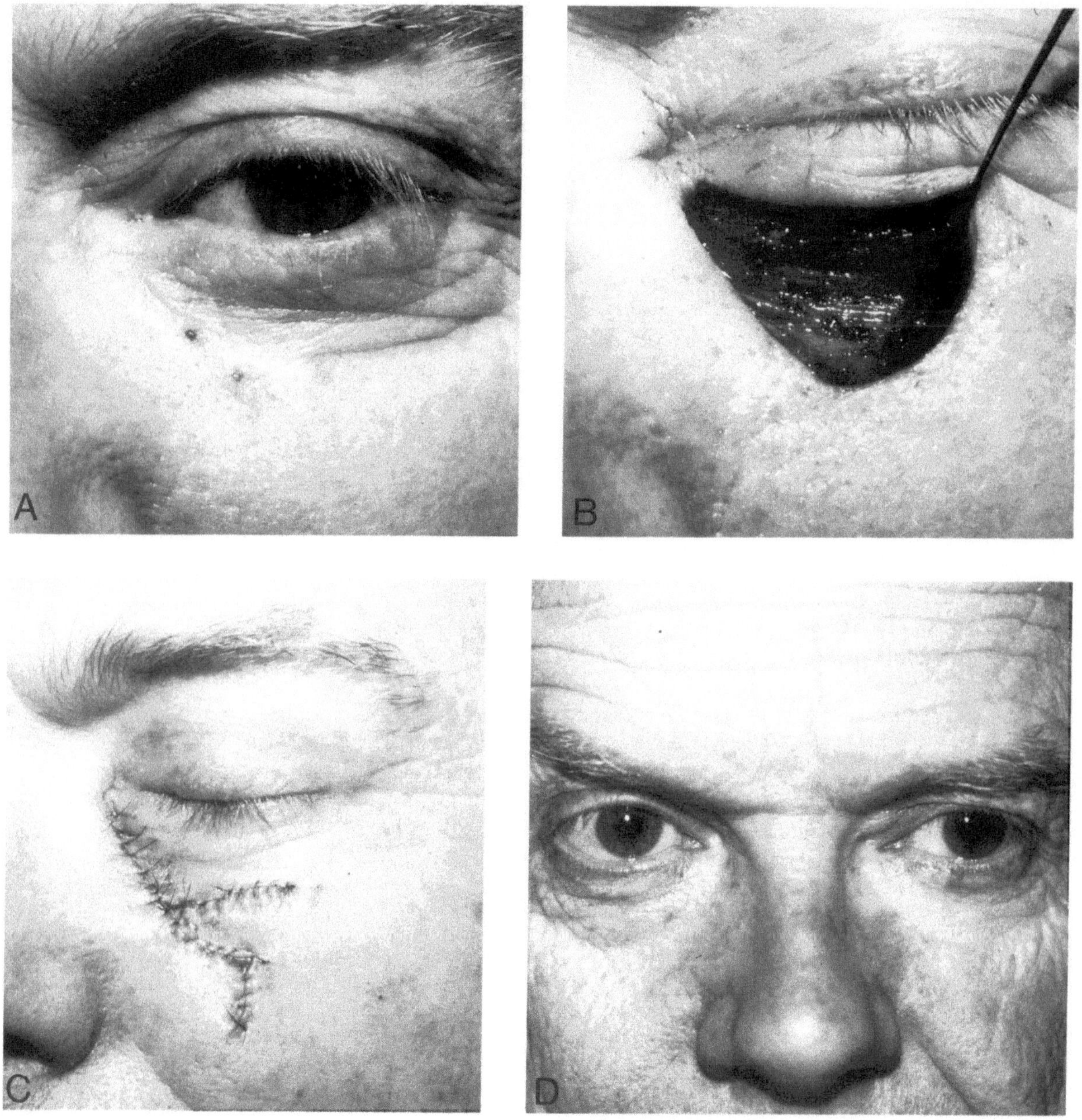

Fig. 5.4 A–D. A "good" aesthetic result. **A** A 56-year-old patient with a BCC of the lower eyelid that has recurred after radiotherapy. **B** The wide excision has included part of the m. orbicularis. **C** Repair with an LLL-flap and primary closure of the medial end of the defect. **D** At 4 years the appearance of the lid is satisfactory but there is asymmetry in relation to the contralateral lid. Therefore, the result is considered "good". Compare with color plate IIB, where a kite flap was used

Fig. 5.5 A–D. A "mediocre" aesthetic result. **A** BCC that has recurred after radiotherapy in a 64-year-old patient. **B** Following excision. **C** Definitive histologic sections revealed an inadequate margin anteriorly. Reexcision was caried out 8 days later and a second full-thickness graft was applied. Intraoperative histology at the initial procedure would have prevented this problem. **D** At 4 years there is a patchwork appearance, and the result is considered "mediocre"

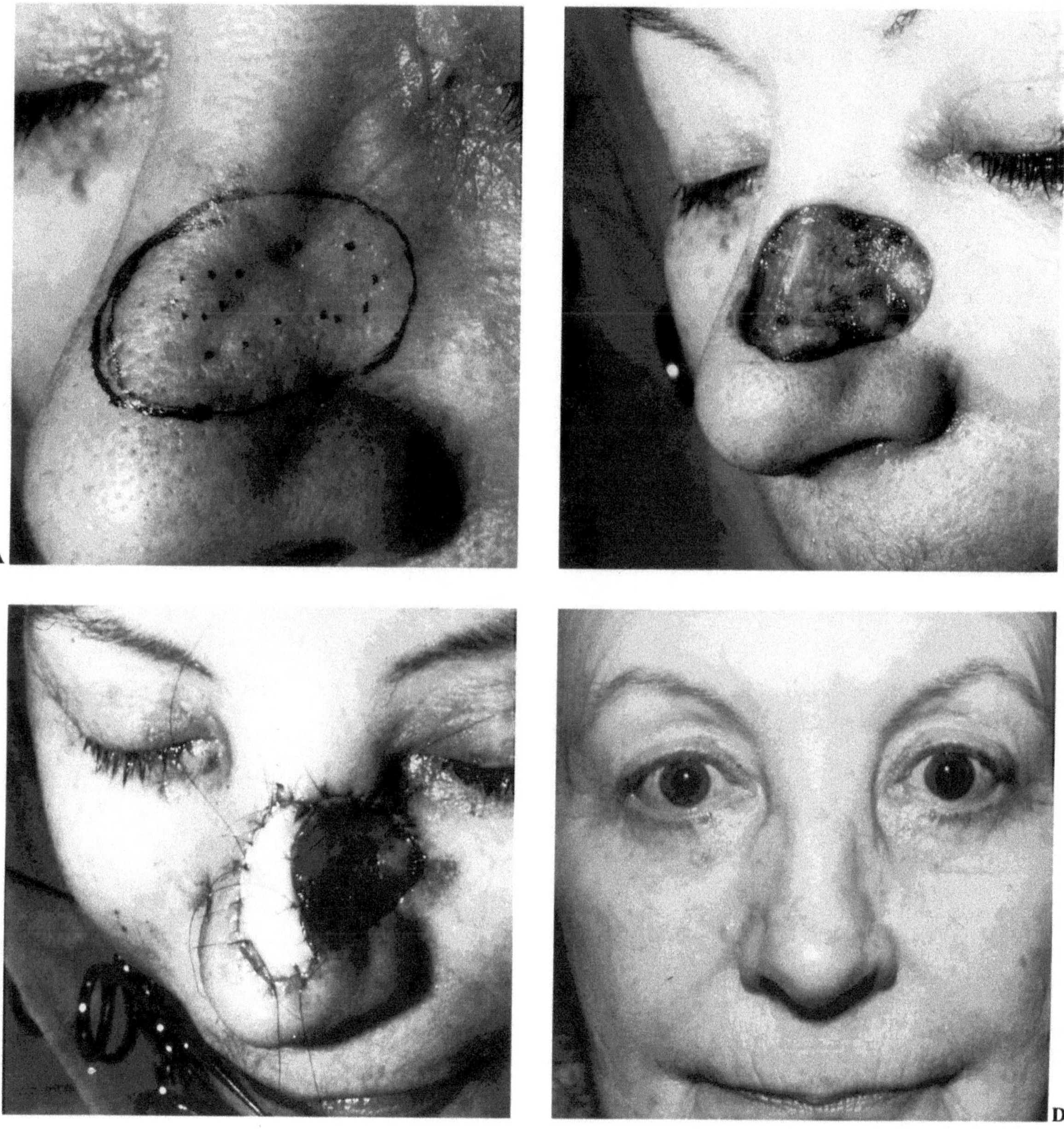

A B C D

Fig. 5.6 A–D. A "mediocre" aesthetic result. **A** A wide, full-thickness excision. The margins are verified intraoperatively. **B** The one-stage repair includes a mucosal flap, a midline forehead flap, and a nasolabial flap. **C** The preoperative appearance of this lesion that had recurred following electrodesiccation. **D** At 8 years the forehead flap is distinctly visible. Although the patient is very pleased, the result is graded "mediocre"

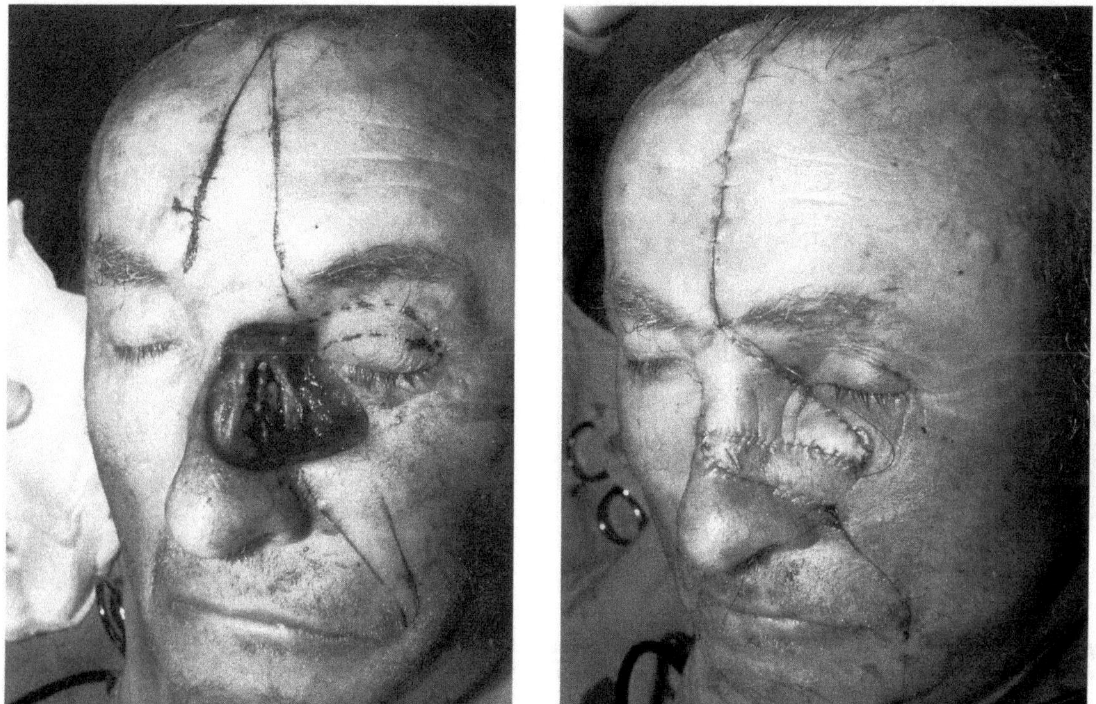
A
B
C
D

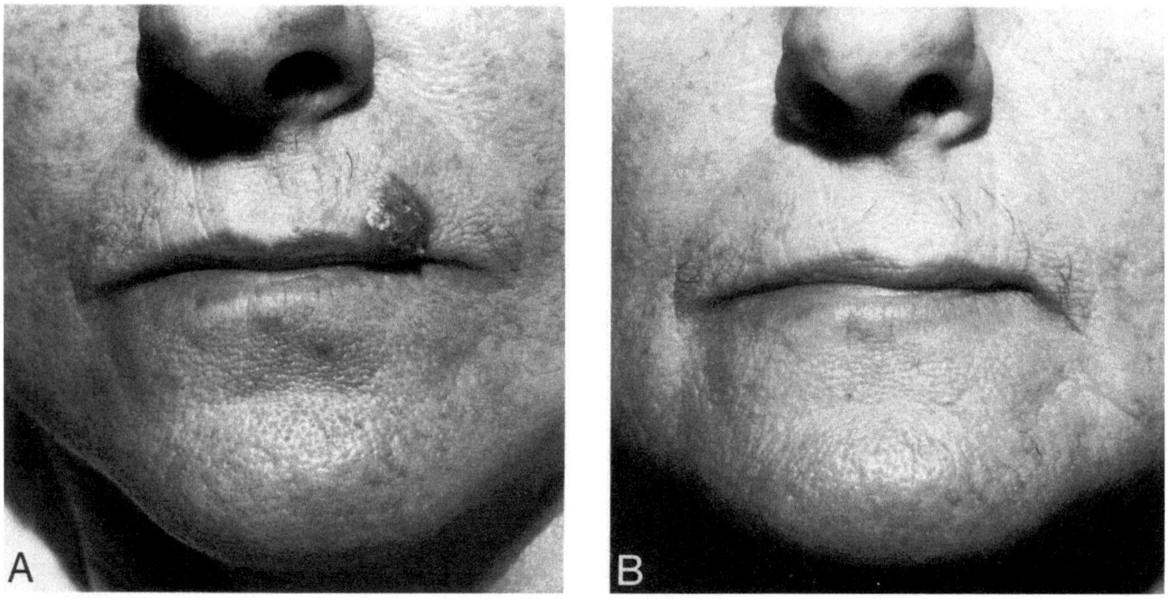

Fig. 5.7 A, B. A "mediocre" aesthetic result. **A** A papulo-pearly BCC in a 68-year-old woman. **B** Three years after wedge resection. The scar is barely visible, but the asymmetry with deviation of the philtrum leads to a grading of "mediocre"

Fig. 5.8 A–D. A "poor" aesthetic result. **A** This 72-year-old patient presents a BCC that has recurred after radiotherapy and has been present for 6 years. **B** A vast resection is carried out. **C** The nostril is reconstructed with a forehead flap and a full-thickness graft is applied to the lip. **D** Appearance at 3 years. The nose is asymmetric, the graft is visible and pulls the lip upward, and the forehead donor site is conspicuous. The result is aesthetically "poor"

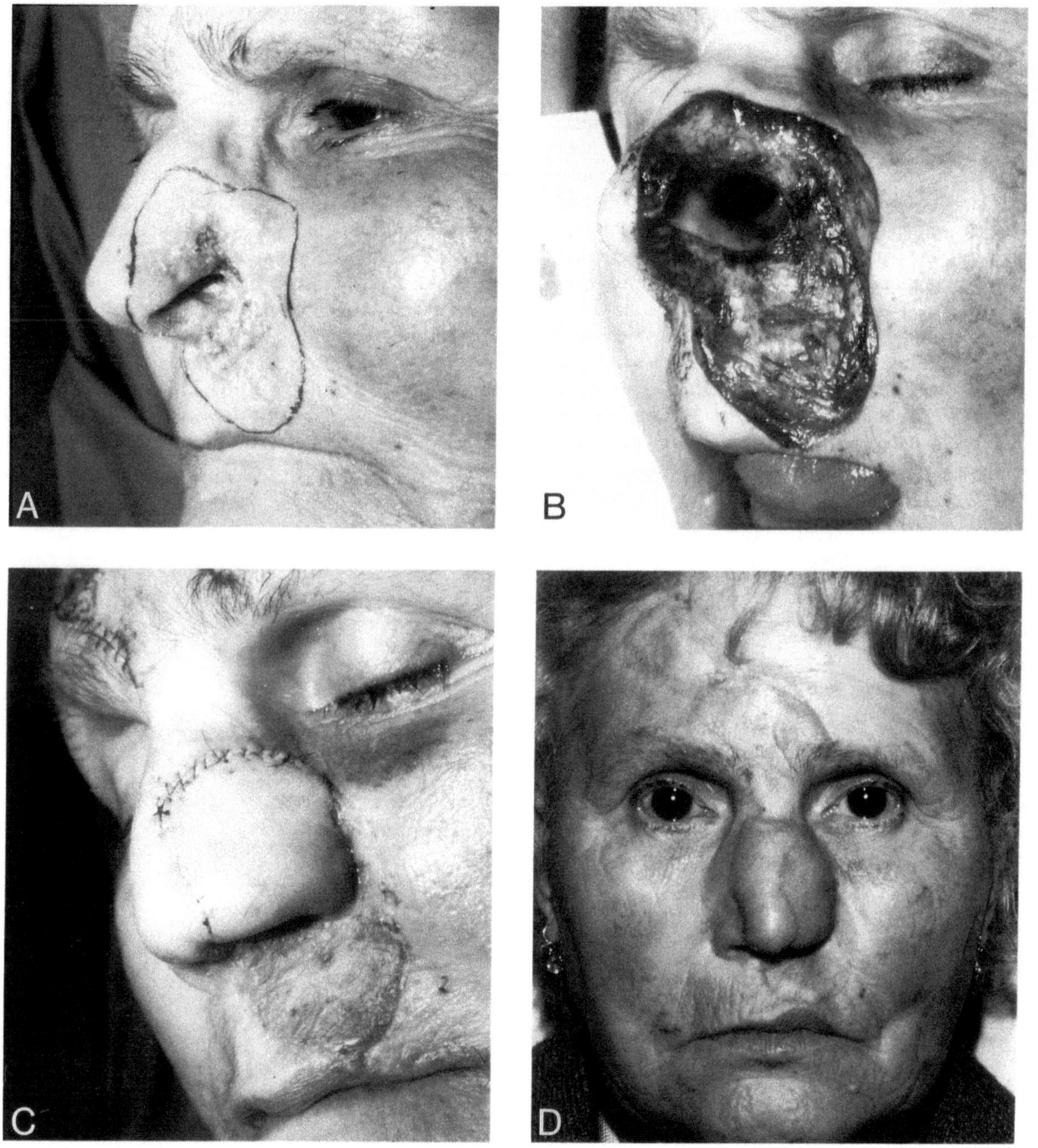

Discussion of the Aesthetic Results

Our classification is debatable, in particular the distinction between 'good' and 'mediocre', i.e., between what is acceptable and what is not. Often the result is imperfect, and yet it would be excessively harsh to classify it as mediocre. The creation of a fifth intermediate category does not appear useful, and basic questioning should be sufficient to tip the balance in one direction or the other.

In general, the patient's judgment coincides with that of the examining surgeon, but striking discordances may occur. The very elegant patient in Fig. 5.3 considered herself multilated and evaluated as poor an objectively excellent result. Inversely, the farmer in Fig. 5.6 thought his result excellent, although it had been judged mediocre by an unbiased observer. The patient in Fig. 5.4 considered his result excellent because there was no visible scar on the operated eyelid. However, he was evaluated as only 'good' because of the asymmetry produced by the opposite lid, which contained excess skin.

Among the excellent results, 6% correspond to lesions situated close to the scalp and repaired by a large flab, with the scars concealed in the hair-bearing skin (Fig. 4.43). On the other hand, the other 94% of excellent aesthetic results were located in the exposed areas of the face. The kite flap of Dufourmentel (Dufourmentel and Talaat 1971) was widely used for the eyelids and the cheeks. The H- and T-flaps were used in the forehead and the frontonasal flap (Marchac 1970) in the nose. All these flaps yielded a large proportion of good results, despite scars that are occasionally quite long. The length of the scar is of secondary importance compared with its fineness and with the overall quality of the repair. The scar should be placed in natural skin folds along anatomic borders without causing distortion. The quality of postoperative care (see p. 19) is important in obtaining a good scar.

Chapter 6 **Indications**

For each patient presenting with a BCC one must choose the treatment that will allow the greatest chances for cure, leave minimal deformity, and be as simple and rapid as possible (Albright 1982).

Our analysis of 225 cases has demonstrated that surgical treatment fulfills these criteria for the great majority of BCCs. The operation is usually undertaken with the patient under local anesthesia and on an outpatient basis; it lasts 30–45 min, and the postoperative course is usually brief and painless. Healing has usually occurred by the 5th or 6th day, when the sutures are removed. By 1 month there is usually minimal deformity, although the final aesthetic result cannot be judged before 6–9 months post-op. The results are good to excellent in 93% of cases, and the cure rate is 97.8% at 3 years.

Advanced age or underlying medical problems are not contraindications to surgery, except in the case of advanced lesions requiring prolonged surgery. For the usual lesions operated with the patient under local anesthesia, surgery is very well tolerated. Although the sutures may even be removed at home, most patients are able to come to the office a week after surgery. This was the case with ten of our patients who were over 90 years old.

This protocol compares very favorably with the inconvenience of numerous treatment sessions for radiotherapy, or with the prolonged healing time required for cryotherapy or electrocoagulation.

Certain lesions appear surgically unfavorable to many dermatologists, especially those of the eyelids, which are often referred for radiotherapy. This may achieve excellent results, but the incidence of loss of the eyelashes appears a significant complication, when one considers that up to one quarter of the width of the lid can be removed without producing deformity. Moreover, most patients present sufficient skin laxity in this region to allow excision and repair of relatively large lesions. Surgical excision can be safely undertaken in close proximity to the lacrimal apparatus, while radiotherapy is not infrequently complicated by stenosis of the canaliculus (Color Plate IIA, p. 109).

Additionally, radiotherapy does not provide histologic verification of eradication of the tumor, recurrences following irradiation are often difficult to detect and to treat, surgical repair is less easy in irradiated tissues and, finally, even mild radiodermatitis presents a risk for the future.

Cryosurgery requires a longer postoperative course and is not simpler to execute than conventional surgery.

Of course we do not maintain that surgery is the only possible therapeutic alternative. In fact, certain patients should preferably be treated using other modalities.

Cryosurgery appears to have three indications:

1. Widespread, superficial, poorly delimited lesions, especially in elderly patients. Conventional surgery would involve a large skin graft which might be poorly tolerated and which often yields a poor aesthetic result.
2. Multiple lesions, usually observed in elderly patients. In such cases surgery is prolonged and often difficult and is likely to result in a mediocre appearence.
3. Small, well-defined lesions of the nose close to the nostril margin. Repair of the nostril margin is difficult since the least irregularity of this delicate structure is visible. The thick dermis in this region favors healing following cryosurgery.

Radiotherapy is useful in avoiding the mutilation that follows excision of massive lesions. In particular, giant

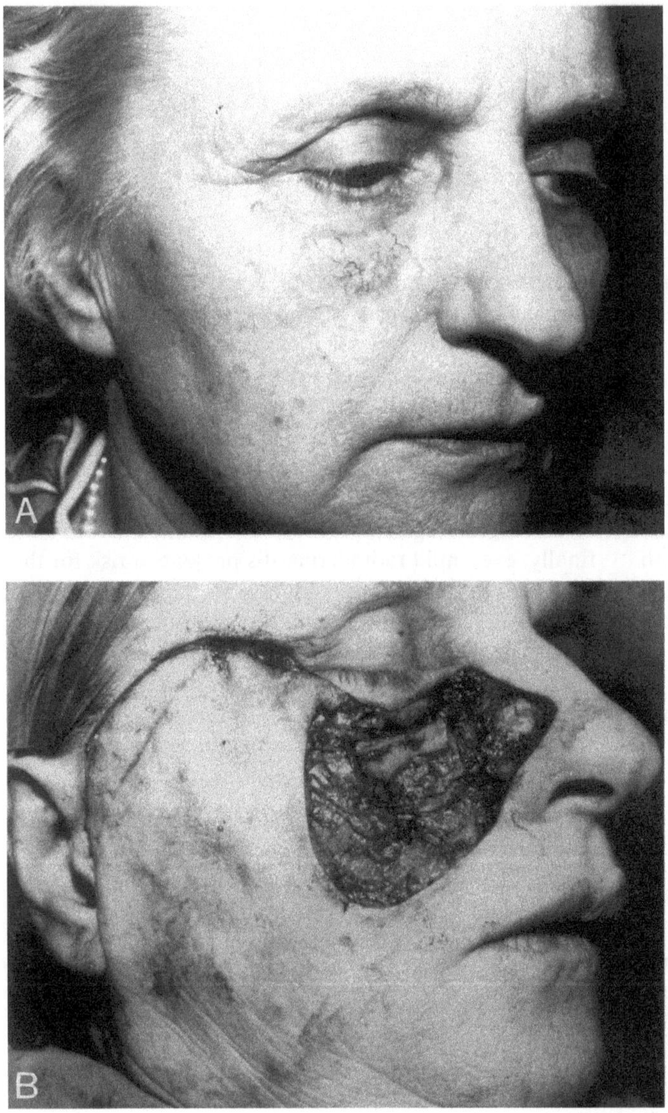

Fig. 6.1 A–F. Untreated lesion of long standing. **A** A 62-year-old patient with a large sclerosing BCC that had been present for 5 years. **B** The excision has exposed the inferior orbital rim. A Mustardé-type cheek flap is raised. **C** The cheek flap is advanced and a forehead flap designed. **D** The forehead flap is inset. Part of the pedicle will be used to resurface the residual defect of the nose. **E** and **F** Result at 13 months. There are no functional problems, but the aesthetic result is mediocre

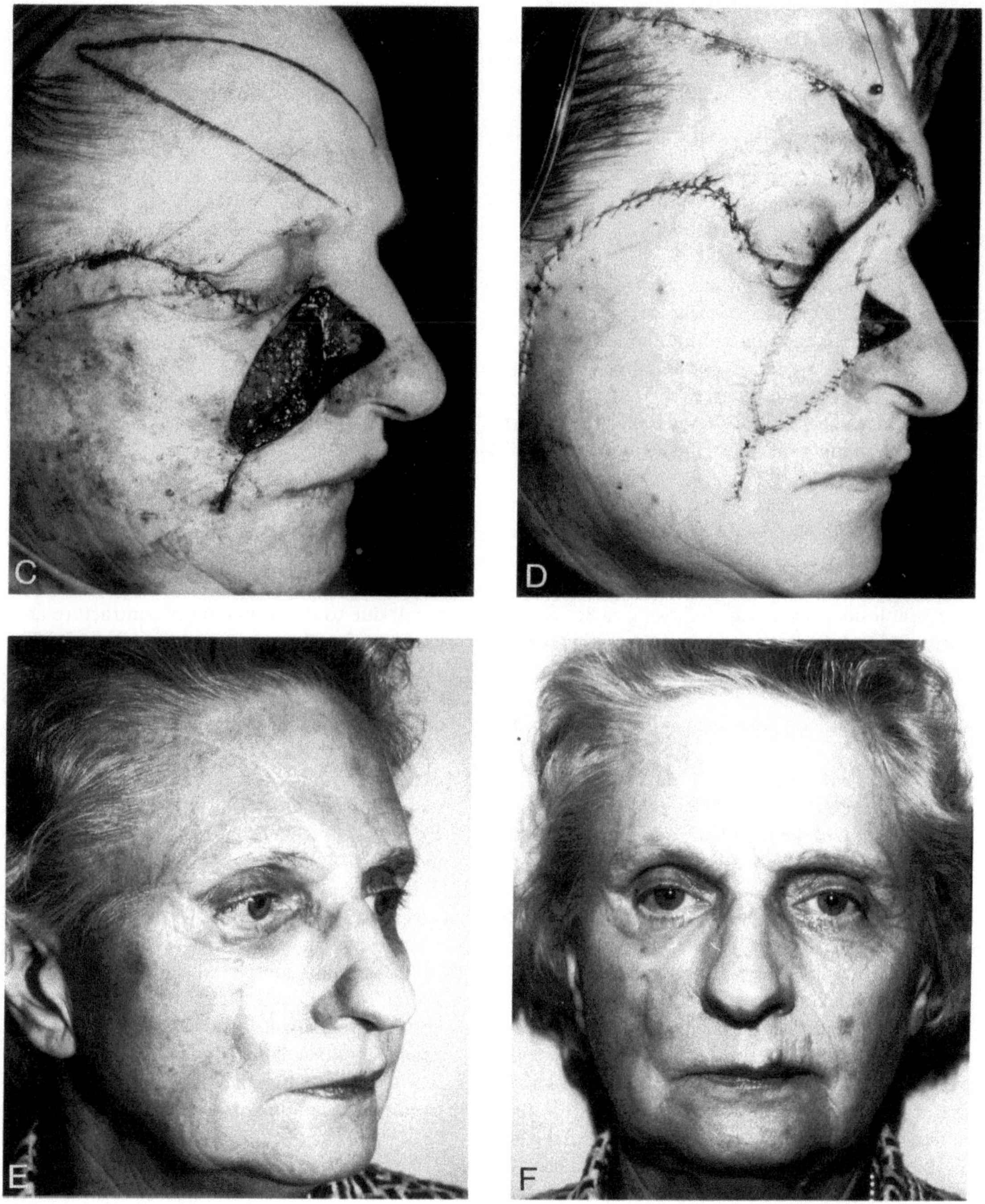
C
D
E
F

BCCs of the nose that would otherwise necessitate amputation can be treated by interstitial irradiation using iridium 192.

If conventional surgery is elected, several questions arise:

1. What will be the extent of the excision?
2. Should intraoperative histology be planned?
3. What is the basic plan for repair?

Theoretically, the *extent of the resection* cannot be evaluated before one has excised to clear margins. However, by drawing a line of excision around the lesion one can estimate the eventual defect and decide whether the repair falls within one's capacities.

The patient is informed of the general protocol, the estimated operating time, and the type of anesthetic planned (see p. 8).

An *intraoperative histologic examination* is planned when the limits of the lesion are poorly defined, as in the following situations:

- Recurrent lesions, especially following radiotherapy
- Poorly defined lesions such as sclerosing BCC or tumors developing in preexisting lesions such as burns or lupus vulgaris
- Anatomically difficult areas such as the medial canthus

The usefulness and validity of intraoperative histology are discussed in Chap. 2.

The final choice of the *technique used for repair* cannot be made before an adequate excision has been carried out. It is not rare to have to change the planned repair during the course of the operation, usually because the defect is larger or shaped differently than had been expected. Once again, the importance of having a complete range of techniques at one's disposal is underlined.

To repair the defect the surgeon selects the procedure that will provide the best aesthetic result, will not produce deformity, and will minimize scars and disparities in texture. Each case is distinguished by the depth of the defect, the elasticity of the surrounding skin, the presence of wrinkles, and the texture, color, and presence of hair in the missing skin. An elliptical excision can be used in areas of good skin laxity. The indications for this technique have been discussed in Chap. 3. It is best avoided where closure must overcome significant tension and in areas where asymmetry may be produced.

When the size or the location of the defect argue against elliptical excision, the choice for repair lies between a skin graft and a flap. The full-thickness skin graft is preferred by many surgeons (Casson 1980; Emmett and O'Rourke 1982; Sundel et al. 1966) who feel it permits easier detection of tumor recurrence. In their view, a flap might conceal recurrence along the deep margin and make the follow-up more difficult.

We do not share this point of view. None of the five recurrences among the 225 lesions (see Chap. 5) occurred at the deep margin; all were located along the lateral margins. This may be due to the fact that we do not hesitate to carry out deep excisions since we are not concerned with preserving a graft bed.

Despite all conceivable precautions, the full-thickness graft carries a risk of failure due even to the smallest hematoma. Although loss is usually partial, this prolongs the postoperative course and compromises the aesthetic result due to the formation of contracture and scar. The graft is often hypo- or hyperpigmented relative to the surrounding tissues and presents differences in texture and vascularity. The graft is often depressed since it carries no subcutaneous tissue to the site of reconstruction. Nevertheless, the full-thickness graft may provide excellent results and become nearly invisible. However, its unpredictability makes it an alternative of last resort, to be used when there is no satisfactory local flap available.

In our view the local flap is the technique of choice; it was used in 57% of our 225 cases. This proportion has been even higher in recent years due to the increasing use of the subcutaneously pedicled kite flap in preference to the full-thickness graft. In each case the best flap is selected to provide good quality coverage with a minimum of scars and distortion.

However, the indications for a local flap may be modified by a number of circumstances:

- *Previous radiotherapy* may increase the risk of flap necrosis. It should be emphasized that skin-graft take may also be jeopardized and that distant flaps are often indicated instead.

- The existence of *scars* secondary to trauma or previous surgery should be ruled out in the region of the planned flap or its pedicle.
- *Tobacco consumption* affects the cutaneous blood supply, and prudence should be exercised in the case of heavy smokers.
- Adjacent *skin laxity* is obviously necessary, as are appropriate color and texture. For example, forehead skin would preferably not be used to resurface an eyelid, nor would a hair-bearing flap be used in a hairless region.

Flap failure must be anticipated, although complete necrosis secondary to inadequate blood supply is rare. We had a single failure in a recent island forehead flap, and we did not observe any complete flap losses in the series of 225 cases. One case of partial necrosis of a nasal flap healed secondarily with satisfactory results. On the other hand, it is not rare to observe minor healing problems at the distal end of the flap where tension is usually maximal and where slight dehiscence may occur. Secondary healing generally leads to satisfactory results.

These problems are unusual, and the great majority of properly planned local flaps heal uneventfully. Certainly, the risk of complications is less for local flaps than for grafts. However, the rate of flap healing is variable, with some flaps nearly invisible after a few weeks and others requiring 6–9 months to stabilize. In either case, the long-term result is usually good.

Occasionally, other techniques are indicated. *Composite grafts* are used (a) to reconstruct the nostril margin using a composite graft from the ear, and (b) to repair an upper eyelid with a graft harvested from the contralateral lid. The most frequently used *distant flap* is the forehead flap, which can be transposed in a single stage as an island flap or in a two-stage procedure, and which is generally used to resurface the nose.

The repair of massive BCCs poses particular problems. In the region of the forehead the frontal bone and dura may be involved. Neurosurgical support must be available if deep involvement is suspected (see Fig. 4.47).

Large lesions of the nose may extend into the nasal fossae and maxillary sinuses. Reconstruction usually requires one flap for the cavity and a second for the surface. Bone grafts are often necessary to reconstitute the bony architecture.

Orbital exenteration may be indicated when the tumor extends into the orbit. In these cases the eyelids must usually be sacrificed and the mutilation is considerable. The orbit may be filled with an m. temporalis flap, which is in turn covered with a skin graft or a forehead flap.

These lesions evolve slowly, over 5–10 years, and many have been neglected by the patients. Since they are painless they may attain considerable size (Fig. 6.1 and Color Plate IB, p. 108). We have seen a rather elegant woman who had hidden a giant BCC beneath a wig, and an engineer who had allowed a tumor to destroy his lower eyelid and the side of his nose over the course of 5 or 6 years.

Chapter 7 Complications of Surgical Treatment

Early Complications

Hemorrhage. Delayed bleeding may develop several hours after surgery with the disappearance of the vasoconstrictive effects of the adrenaline. In general, this is easily controlled with local compression, and reoperation is rarely required.

The risk of hemorrhage is reduced by (a) discontinuing aspirin at least 10 days prior to surgery, (b) verifying that coagulation tests are normal in doubtful cases, and (c) decreasing or stopping treatment with anticoagulants several days before surgery, with the agreement of the treating physician. If this is impossible, then surgical treatment must be deferred.

Infection. In the early postoperative period, erythema, swelling, and pain signal infection. This may resolve following the application of alcohol compresses or Hexomedine transcutaneous (Théraplix Laboratories), but more often an abscess will form. Healing occurs following evacuation of the collection.

Antibiotic therapy is reserved for infections seen very early and those which diffuse or fail to resolve with other measures. A culture should be taken before therapy is begun.

Prevention of infection depends on aseptic operative technique. Unfortunately, there are often sources of contamination or small infections near the operative site. These must be carefully disinfected during preparation of the face.

The rarity of infection is remarkable in this area where natural orifices abound. It can be explained by the rich vascularity of the face.

Dehiscence. This complication may be the result of (a) poorly-tied knots and (b) excessive tension on the wound, with the sutures cutting through the tissues. Knots made with certain types of suture, especially monofilament nylon, show a disturbing tendency to untie, and three or four knots should always be placed when these materials are used.

Excessive tension must obviously be avoided. Various measures include (a) taking up tension in the deep plane, (b) using U-type far-near-near-far stitches to approximate the edges, and (c) placing a running subcuticular suture, which provides good dermal approximation but which must be completed, when tension exists, with a running suture or with fine simple sutures. These are removed early and replaced with adhesive strips.

When dehiscence has resulted from excessive tension and impaired viability of the margins, no attempt is made to close the wound. Superfluous suture material is removed and adhesive strips are applied at either end of the area of separation while waiting for secondary healing to occur.

In unusual cases where dehiscence is early and the wound clean, a local flap may be used to obtain closure without tension.

In most instances involving small areas of dehiscence, secondary healing yields an acceptable scar.

Partial or Total Flap Necrosis. Flap viability may be compromised either by intrinsic vascular insufficiency or by compression of the pedicle.

Occasionally, especially in flaps with narrow pedicles, complete flap failure is evident. A white flap indicates arterial failure. If there is no compression or torsion of the pedicle there is little to be done. If the flap is blue, then venous return is inadequate, and the wound may be partially opened to allow bleeding from the margin, or leaches may be applied for 24–48 h. If the flap appears compromised from the outset, and especially in the case of white flaps, the skin may be salvaged and applied as a full-thickness graft.

More often, the viability of the flap is uncertain, especially in its distal portion. The color is unsatisfactory and the flap is mottled. In these cases a wait-and-see attitude is indicated and the sutures are left in place. Sometimes the flap goes on to heal, while in others demarcation occurs between the viable and necrotic zones. When this is clearly established, by 10–15 days, one should excise the necrotic area without waiting for spontaneous separation. This saves time and decreases the chance of infection. One should not hesitate to carry out a wide excision; all doubtful areas should be excised to viable, bleeding tissue.

The wound is cleaned daily with a disinfectant solution and dressed with tulle gras. Secondary healing will occur and the scar can be revised at around 6 months.

Partial or Total Graft Loss. Removal of the tie-over dressing on the 5th day is usually associated with some anxiety, since one can never be sure that the graft has taken. Occasionally, one is disappointed to observe dark blue areas under the graft, or even a graft that is blue throughout. At this stage, on the 5th or 6th day, it is too late to save those areas of the graft that have been lifted by hematoma.

In rare cases where a large hematoma has resulted in complete loss of the graft, débridement and immediate regrafting may be undertaken. More often there is partial loss, and conservative débridement is carried out to allow secondary healing to occur.

Prevention of this complication is based on hemostasis and imobilization of the graft, both discussed on p. 21.

Late Complications

Hypertrophic Scars. These may occur anywhere, through they are more frequent in certain areas, such as at the border of the mandible. After several weeks the healing incision becomes hypertrophic, erythematous, and pruritic. A wait-and-see attitude is indicated, and occasionally massages with hydrocortisone cream may be prescribed. The problem usually subsides after several months (see p. 19).

Scar contracture, especially in the eyelids or perioral region, may be corrected with a procedure such as Z-plasty. The tension on the scar causes the hypertrophic reaction, which resolves when the tension is released.

Compression therapy is very effective for hypertrophic scars, although it may be difficult to use in the face.

Flaps. The "trapdoor phenomenon" is manifested by chronic edema of the flap with peripheral contracture of the scar (Fig. 4.13). Massage, compression, and time will improve the problem as the lymphatic circulation is reestablished. This problem will rarely develop if the flap has been carefully inset under mild tension and the wound has been closed in two layers.

Telangiectasia occasionally appear on the distal ends of flaps and in adjacent skin. Although the pathogenesis is unclear, they may be effectively treated using fine electrocoagulation or laser.

Grafts. Pigment changes often appear late in the course of healing of skin grafts. Although full-thickness grafts usually conserve the pigmentation of the donor site, they may sometimes undergo hyperpigmentation. This is usually seen after exposure to the sun during the first month and may be prevented by avoiding such exposure and using sunscreens. Once established, graft hyperpigmentation may resolve spontaneously after several years.

Deformities. Various deformities may be observed following the use of any of these repair methods; they include:

- Misalignment of the skin edges, producing a step deformity
- Excess thickness, especially in flaps
- Depression at the site of a widened scar or a skin graft (Fig. 5.5)
- Distortion of facial landmarks, such as elevation of a nostril, or eversion or inversion of a lip or an eyelid (Fig. 7.1)

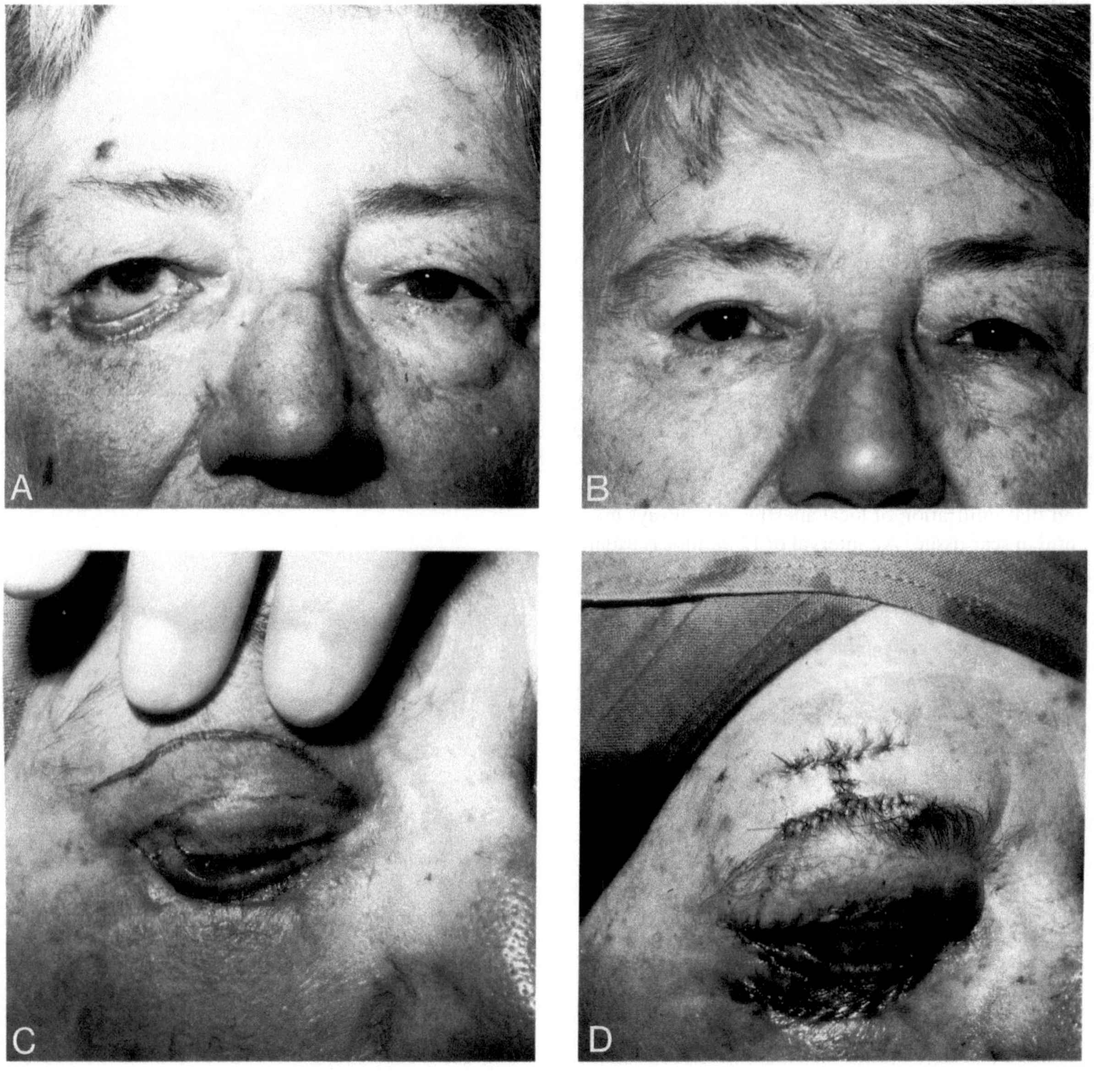

Fig. 7.1 A–D. Ectropion. **A** This 75-year-old patient was referred for correction of an ectropion that had developed after excision of a BCC of the lower lid. **B** At 2 years the lid has maintained satisfactory height. **C** and **D** Correction was obtained with a laterally based flap transposed from the upper lid to the lower. The frontal H-flap was used following the excision of a second BCC

In some instances the deformity is not apparent at rest, and the disruption of normal skin folds is noted only during smiling or grimacing. This is particularly true in the nasolabial fold, and one should avoid placing flaps across this area (see Fig. 4.9). This is also the case with the lateral nose, which wrinkles during smiling.

Revisions

The cardinal rule governing revisions is that one should never hurry to reoperate. Only in unusual cases involving a functional disturbance such as ectropion should reoperation be carried out quickly.

In general, revision is not planned until 6–9 months have elapsed and the final result can be evaluated. A simple scar revision, a local flap or a skin graft may be required at this stage. The presence of existing scars must be carefully taken into account, and it should be remembered that infiltration of local anesthesia is always more painful in scar tissue. An interval of 12 months is usually required before the result of the revision can be assessed.

Conclusion

At the present time the surgical treatment of BCCs of the face is simple and safe thanks to progress in the techniques of plastic surgery. This safety and this simplicity are possible only in the hands of a trained operator, in part because of the complex structure of the face.

Dermatologic training, which allows one to recognize the lesion and to distinguish its limits, and surgical competence in resection and reconstruction are desirable for the treatment of these lesions.

We hope to have provided, in these few pages, information useful to those interested in these very frequent tumors.

Color Plates

Color Plate I

A An H-flap of the forehead in a 68-year-old-man. At 3 months the result is "excellent" (see evaluation of aesthetic results, p. 87)

B Ulcerated, untreated lesion in a 41-year-old woman. The resection included nasal bone and an extension of tumor into the left orbit. At 1 year repair with an island forehead flap has produced a mediocre aesthetic result

C An 89-year-old patient presenting with a second recurrence of a BCC after electrodesiccation and cryotherapy. A frontonasal flap mobilizes the entire nasal cover on a narrow pedicle. At 1 year the result is judged "excellent"

D A large recurrent lesion 8 years following excision and skin grafting in an 86-year-old man. A large cheek-advancement flap allows repair of the defect. At 6 months the result is excellent

Color Plate II

A This BCC is located near the inferior lacrimal point, which is sacrificed by a wide excision. The lid is closed primarily with the aid of a lateral cantholysis. A silicone catheter is introduced into the remaining canaliculus. At 3 months there is no tearing and the aesthetic result is judged "excellent"

B This BCC of the lower lid in a 66-year-old man is excised and resurfaced with a kite flap. Sixteen months later symmetry has been preserved and the scars are hidden in natural folds. The aesthetic result is "excellent"

C This 43-year-old patient presented with a recurrent BCC following cryotherapy. A wedge resection would have deformed the lip. A kite flap is combined with a flap of mucosa to reconstruct the defect. At 6 months there is no deformity and the scar is beginning to fade

D An ulcerated BCC that has developed at the site of an old scar in a 63-year-old man. An LLL-flap is used to repair the defect; the area of depressed scar is excised along with the dog-ear created by transposition of the flap. At 4 months the scar is beginning to fade and there is no deformity. The final result will most likely be "good" since the scar will remain somewhat visible

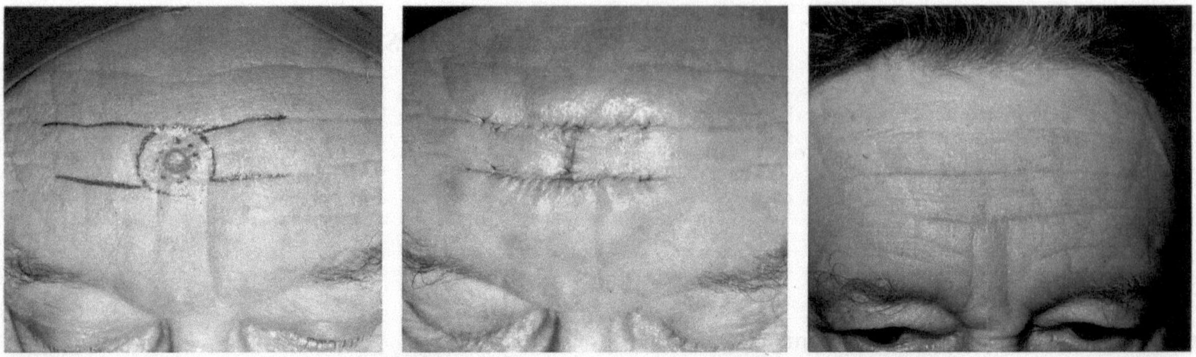

IA

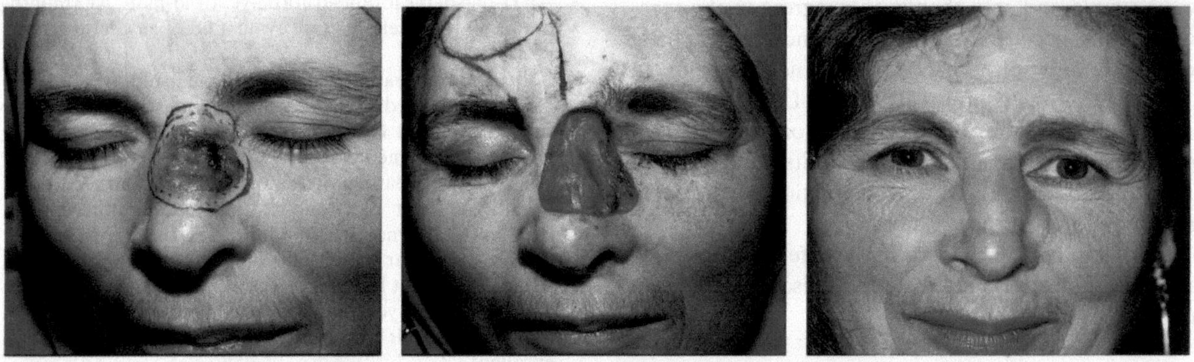

IB

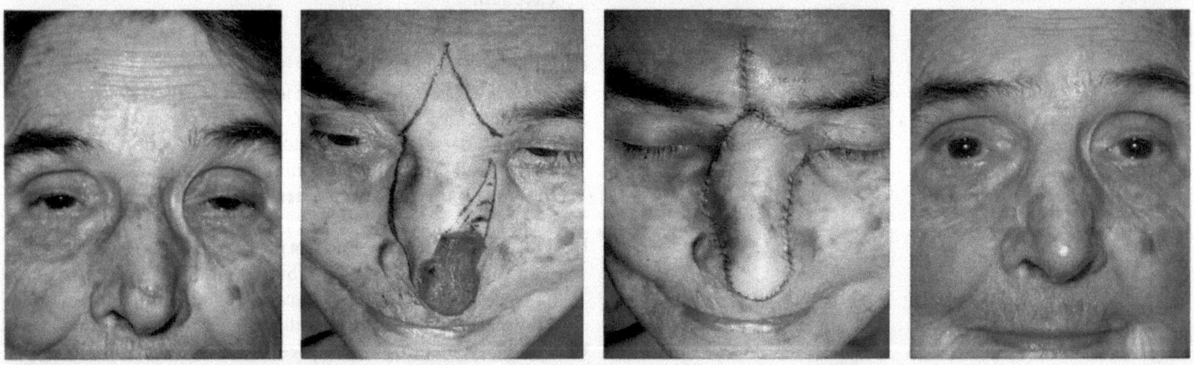

IC

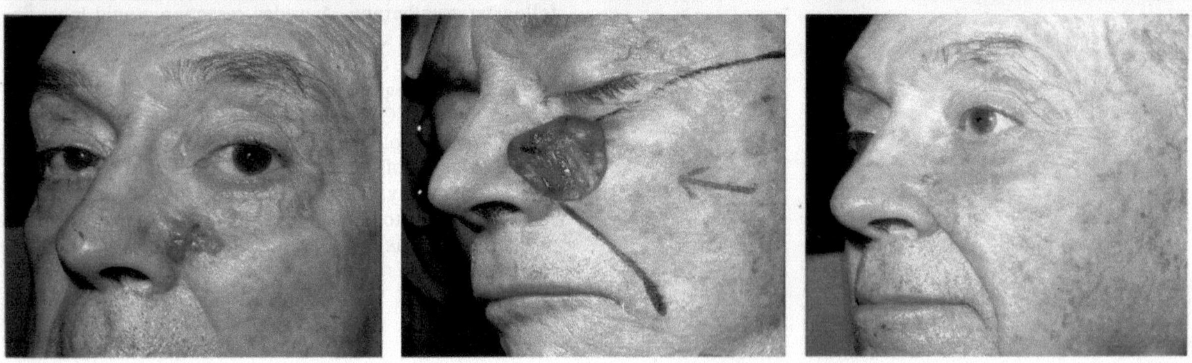

ID

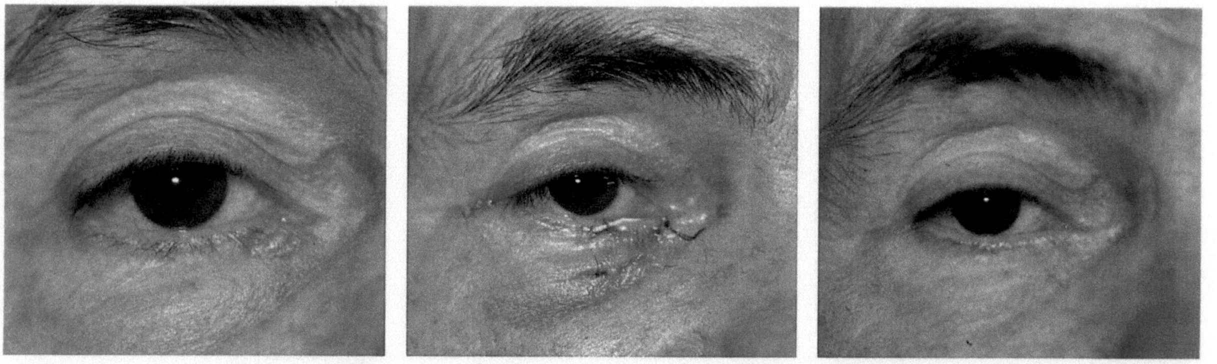
IIA

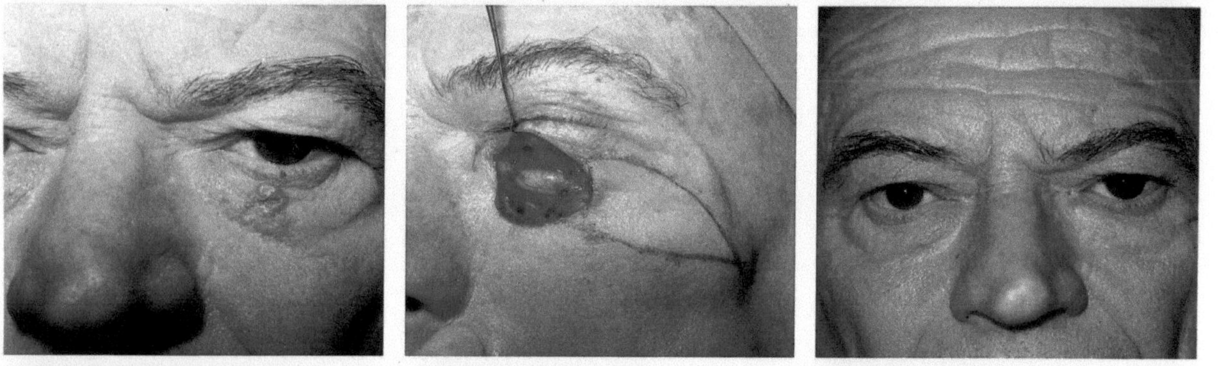
IIB

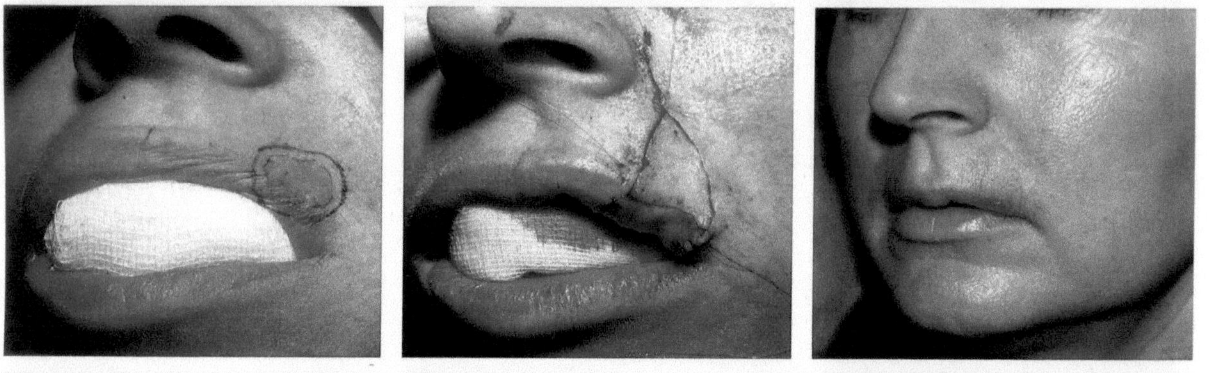
IIC

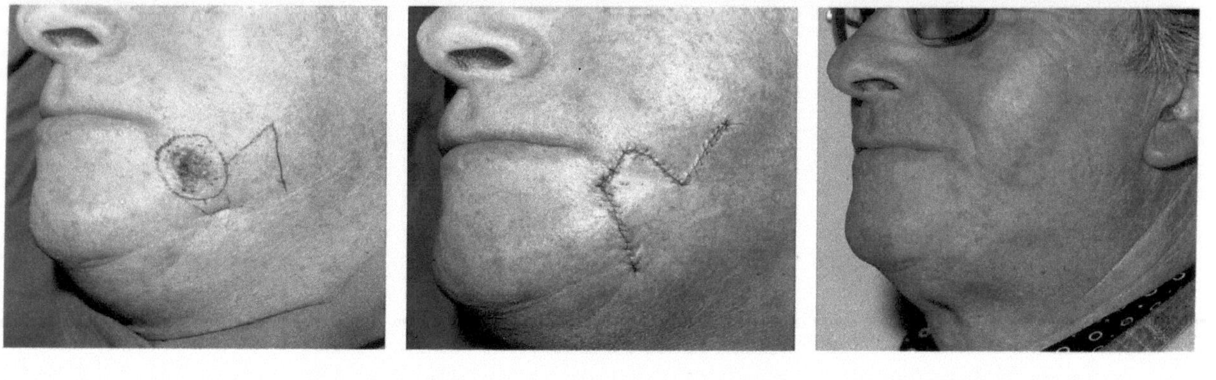
IID

References

Abide JM, Nahai F, Bennett R (1984) The meaning of surgical margins. Plast Reconstr Surg 73:492–496

Albright SD (1982) Treatment of skin cancer using multiple modalities. Am Acad Dermatol 7:143–171

Amalric R, Calas E, Seigle L, Join P (1974) Indications et résultats de l'électronthérapie dans les épithéliomas cutanés. Bull Soc F Derm Syph 81:66–68

Baker PB, Bergren R (1983) Metastatic basal cell carcinoma: review and report of a case. Ann Plast Surg 11:428

Bart R, Kopf AW (1979) Techniques of biopsy of cutaneous neoplasms. J Dermatol Surg Oncol 5:979–987

Bart R, Schrager D (1978) Scalpel excision of basal cell carcinoma. Arch Dermatol 114:739

Belisario JC (1964) An appraisal of therapeutic methods for skin carcinomas by scalpel or electrosurgery, ionizing radiation, electrochemosurgery, and local chemotherapy. Acta Derm Venereol (Stockh) 44:1–34

Binstock JH et al. (1981) Large aggressive basal cell carcinomas of the scalp. J Dermatol Surg Oncol 7:565–569

Biro L, Price E, Mac Williams P (1975) Basal cell carcinoma in office practice. NY State J Med 75:1427–1433

Burg G, Hirsch RD, Konz B, Braun-Falco O (1975) Histographic surgery. Accuracy of visual assessment of the margins of basal cell epithelioma. J Dermatol Surg Oncol 1:21

Casson P (1980) Basal cell carcinoma. Clinics Plast Surg 7:301–311

Ceilley R, Anderson RL (1978) Microscopically controlled excision of malignant neoplasms on and around eyelids followed by immediate surgical reconstruction. J Dermatol Surg Oncol 4:55–62

Chernosky ME (1978) Squamous cell and basal cell carcinomas: preliminary study of 3817 primary skin cancers. South Med J 71:802–806

Curry MD, Montgomery H, Winkelmann RK (1971) Giant basal cell carcinoma. Arch Dermatol 113:316–319

Degos R (1953) Dermatologie. Flammarion, Paris

Degos R (1958) Les cancers de la peau. Presse médicale 66:916–918

Dellon LA (1985) Histologic study of recurrent basal cell carcinoma. Plast Reconstr Surg 75:853–859

Dellon LA, Potvin C et al. (1975) Immunobiology of skin cancer. Plast Reconstr Surg 55:341–354

Dellon LA, De Silva S, Connolly M, Ross A (1985) Prediction of recurrence in incompletely excised basal cell carcinoma. Plast Reconstr Surg 75:860–871

Deutsch HL, Orentreich N (1979) Treatment of small external cancers of the nose. Ann Plast Surg 3:567–571

Dufourmentel C, Talaat SM (1971) The kite flap. Transactions Fifth Int Congress. Plast Reconstr Surg. Melbourne Butterworth, 1123

Duperrat B (1959) Précis de dermatologie. Masson, Ed., Paris, 758–781

Dvoretzky I, Fischer BK, Haker O (1978) Mutilating basal cell epithelioma. Arch Dermatol 114:239–240

Eade G (1974) Basal cell carcinoma. JAMA 33:229

Eckhoff NL (1951) Recurrent, multiple, and metastasising basal cell carcinoma. Br J Plast Surg 3:264–281

Elton RF (1975) Cryosurgery of difficult basal cell epitheliomas. Cutis 16:474–476

Emmett A, O'Rourke M (1982) Malignant skin tumors. Churchill Livingstone, 1 vol, 225

Epstein E (1973) How accurate is the visual assessment of basal cell carcinoma? Br J Dermatol 89:37

Epstein E (1973) Value of follow-up after treatment of basal cell carcinoma. Arch Dermatol 108:798

Epstein E (1974) Cosmetic results after treatment of basal cell carcinoma. Cutis 14:825

Epstein E (1975) Basal cell epithelioma: treat on sight. Int J Dermatol 14:263

Epstein E (1977) Curettage-electrodesiccation vs surgical excision. Arch Dermatol 113:1729

Epstein E, Epstein E Jr (1979) Techniques in skin surgery. Philadelphia. Lea & Febiger

Epstein N (in Epstein E) (1970) Skin surgery. 3rd Ed. Springfield, IL, Charles C Thomas Publisher, 266

Farmer ER, Helwig EB (1980) Metastasic basal cell carcinoma. Cancer 46:748

Freeman RG, Knox JM, Heaton CL (1964) Treatment of skin cancer: a statistical study of 1341 skin tumors comparing results obtained with irradiation, surgery, and curettage followed by electrodesiccation. Cancer 17:535–538

Gage AA (1975) Cryosurgery for difficult problems in cutaneous cancer. Cutis 16:465–470

Godding C, White G, Yatsuhashi M (1965) Significance of marginal extension in excised basal cell carcinoma. New Engl J Med 273:923

Goldberg L, Stal S, Spira M (1983) Recognition and treatment of recurrent baso-cell carcinoma. Ann Plast Surg 11:313

Gormley D (1987) Aggressive basal cell carcinomas. Arch Dermatol 114:782–783

Griffith Mc Kinney (1973) Appraisal of treatment of basal cell carcinoma. Plast Reconstr Surg 51:565

Guiot-Tabernat N (1985) Bulletin de la Société Française de Cancerologie Privée. No 11

Hayes H (1972) Basal cell carcinoma. Plast Reconstr Surg 30:273

Herbert DC, Degens J (1975) Nasolateral subcutaneous pedicle flaps. Br J Plast. Surg 28:90

Jackson R (1973) Basal cell carcinoma, 435 cases. J Surg Oncol 5:431

Jackson R (1974) Why do basal cell carcinomas reccur – or not – following treatment? J Surg Oncol 6:245

Jackson R, Adams RH (1973): Horrifying basal cell carcinoma: a study of 33 cases and a comparison with 435 non-horror cases and a report on four metastatic cases. J Surg Oncol 5:431–463

Jansen GT (1976) Treatment of basal cell epitheliomas and actinic keratoses: JAMA 235:1152–1154

Kalis B, Cavenelle F, L'Huillier F, Triller R (1984) Notre experience des traitements des épithéliomas cutanés par cryochirurgie, de 1981 à 1983. Ann Derm Vener 111:948

Knox JM, Freeman RG, Duncan WC, Heaton CL (1967) Treatment of skin cancer. South Med J 60:241–246

Kopf AW, Bart RS (1975) Skin tumor conference No 3. Recurring basal cell carcinoma following Mohs' surgery. J Dermatol Surg 1:13–15

Kopf AW, Bart RS (1977) Curettage electro-electrodessication treatment of basal cell carcinoma. Arch Dermatol 113:439

Koplin L, Zarem HA (1980) Recurrent basal cell carcinoma. A review concerning the incidence, behavior and management of recurrent basal cell carcinoma. Plast Reconstr Surg 65:656

Lagrot F, Greco J, Coriat P, Bensoussan H, Py N (1956) Traitement réparateur des cancers cutanés de la face et du cuir chevelu. Ann Chir Plast 1:91–116

Lauritzen R, Johnson R, Spratt J (1965) Pattern of recurrence in basal cell carcinoma. Surgery 57:813

Leider J (1980) The rampant basal cell carcinoma; report and lessons of a case. J Dermatol Surg Oncol 6:192–195

Leroux R (1931) Technique nouvelle pour examens histologiques rapide. Bull du Cancer 20:698

Macomber WB, Wanger MKH, Sullivan JG (1959) Cutaneous epithelioma. Plast Reconstr Surg 24:545

Maillard G, Montandon D (1982) The Washio tempororetroauricular flap: its use in 20 patients. Plast Reconstr Surg 70:550–559

Marchac D (1970) Lambeau de rotation fronto-nasal. Ann Chir Plast 5:44–49

Marchac D (1972) Les épithéliomas cutanés des sujets de moins de 40 ans. Nouv Presse Med 1, no 45

Marchac D, Alkhateb B (1974) Les résultats à distance du lambeau fronto-nasal. Ann Chir Plast 19:335–338

Marchac D, Duport G (1980) Résultats carcinologiques et esthétiques du traitement chirurgical de 138 épithéliomas baso-cellulaires. Ann Chir Plast 15:127–134

Marchac D, Larregue M (1986) L'expansion cutanée par implant gonflable. Annales de Dermatologie et de Vénérologie 113:329–337

Mehta H (1979) Surgical management of carcinoma of eyelids and periorbital skin. Br J Ophtalmol 63:578–585

Mohs FE (1976) Chemosurgery for skin cancer. Arch Derm 112:211

Mohs FE (1978) Tendency of fluorouracil to conceal deep foci of invasive basal cell carcinoma. Arch Derm 114:1021

Mohs FE (1978a) Chemosurgery: microscopically controlled surgery for skin cancer – past, present and future. J Dermatol Surg Oncol 4:41–54

Mohs FE (1978b) Chemosurgery, microscopically controlled surgery of skin cancer. Springfield, IL, Charles C Thomas, Publisher

Montes LF, Parker JM (1977) Punch excision technique for removing basal cell epithelioma. Geriatrics 30:414–416

Moore J (1971) Treatment of cicatrizing basal cell carcinoma. Plast Reconstr Surg 47:371

Mora RG, Robins P (1978) Basal cell carcinoma in the center of the face: the special diagnostic, prognostic and therapeutic considerations. J Dermatol Surg Oncol 4:315

Moscona R, Pnini A, Hirshowitz B (1983) In favor of healing by secondary intention after excision of medial canthal basal cell carcinoma. Plast Reconstr Surg 71:189–195

Murray JE, Klein E (1971) Plastic surgical treatment of facial skin cancer. J Surg Oncol 3:269–286

Mustardé J (1966) In: "Repair and reconstruction in the orbital region." Livingstone, Edinburgh, vol 1, p. 125, p. 382

Nevrkla E, Newton KA (1974) A survey of the treatment of 200 cases of basal cell carcinoma (1959–1966). Br J Dermatol 91:429–433

Paletta FW (1977) In "Tumors of the skin". Reconstructive Plastic Surgery. Ed J Converse, Saunders Philadelphia, 2917

Pascal R, Hobby L, Lattres R, Crikelair G (1968) Prognosis of incompletely excised versus completely excised basal cell carcinoma. Plast Reconstr Surg 41:328

Payne JW, Duke JR, Butner R, Eifrig DE (1969) Basal cell carcinoma of the eyelids. Arch Ophthalmol 81:553–558

Pierquin B, Bailler F, Dupre MD (1977) Place de la radiothérapie dans les cancers cutanés. Sem Hop Paris 53:258–260

Pillsbury D (1956) Dermatology. Saunders, Philadelphia 1141–1152

Pinkus H (1966) The borderline between cancer and non cancer. In: Yearbook of Dermatology 67

Plaza de la R, Rodriguez E, Castillo E (1983) Two cases of nevoid basal cell carcinoma syndrome. Plast Reconstr Surg 71:114–119

Popkin GL, Bart RS (1975) Excision versus curettage and electrodesiccation as dermatology office procedures for the treatment of basal-cell carcinomas. J Dermatol Surg Oncol 1:33–35

Porte A, Molle B. Zumer L, Mayer G, Baux S (1979) Résultats du traitement de 250 épithéliomas cutanés. Ann Chir Plast 24:3, 253

Radovan C (1984) Tissue expansion in soft-tissue reconstruction. Plast Reconstr Surg 74:482

Rakofsky SI (1973) The adequacy of the surgical excision of basal cell carcinoma. Ann Ophtalmol 5:596–600

Rank BK, Wakefield AF (1959) Surgery of basal cell carcinoma. Br J Surg 45:531

Reymann F (1972) A follow-up study of treatment of basal cell carcinoma with 5-fluorouracil ointment. Dermatologica 144:205–208

Reymann F (1980) Basal cell carcinoma of the skin; recurrence rate after different types of treatment. A review. Dermatologica 161:217–226

Riberti C, Fasano D, Tirone L, Cavalca D (1983) A propos des épithéliomas baso-cellulaires multifocaux: l'importance de la région temporale. Ann Chir Plast Esth 3, vol 28, 255

Riefkohl R, Wittels B, Mc Carthy K (1984) Metastatic basal cell carcinoma. Ann Plast Surg 13:525–528

Rintala A (1971) Surgical therapy of basal cell carcinoma – correlation of the macroscopic and microscopic control of excision with recurrence. Scand J Plast Reconstr Surg 5:87

Robins P, Ablom M (1975) Recurrent basal cell carcinoma in young women. J Dermatol Surg Oncol 1:49

Robins P, Pollack SV, Robinson JK (1979) Immediate repair of wounds following operations by Mohs' fresh-tissue technique. J Dermatol Surg Oncol 5:329–336

Robinson JK, Pollack SV, Robins P (1980) Invasion of cartilage by basal cell carcinoma. J Am Acad Dermatol 2:499–505

Rogers M (1980) Management of common skin tumors. Med J Aust 2:239–243

Sakura C, Calamel P (1979) Comparison of treatment modalities for recurrent basal cell carcinoma. Plast Reconstr Surg 63

Salasche SJ; Amonette RA (1981) Morpheaform basal-cell epitheliomas: study of subclinical extensions in a series of 51 cases. J Dermatol Surg Oncol 7:387–393

Shanoff LB, Spira M, Hardy SB (1967) Statistical approach to rational treatment of basal cell carcinoma. Plast Reconstr Surg 39:619

Smith JM, Irons GB (1983), Metastatic basal cell carcinoma: review of the literature and report of 3 cases. Ann Plast Surg 11:551

Smith JW (1960) The anatomical and physiologic acclimatization of tissue transplanted by the lip switch technique. Plast Reconstr Surg 76:40

Song R, Ling J, Wang G, Yang R (1982) One-stage reconstruction of the nose in "Clinics in Plastic Surgery". Saunders, Philadelphia, vol 9, no 1

Sundel B, Gylling H, Soivio R (1966) Treatment of basal cell carcinoma by plastic surgery. Acta Chir Scand 131:249

Taylor G, Barisoni D (1973) Ten years' experience in the surgical treatment of basal cell carcinoma. Brit J Surg 60:522

Tessier P (1974) Platysma flap. Personal communication

Tromovitch TA, Stegman SJ (1978) Microscopic controlled excision of cutaneous tumors. Cancer 41:653–658

Waller G, Weidenbecher M (1977) Recurrent basal cell carcinoma of the facial region – a clinico-pathological challenge. Arch Otorhinolaryngol 215:61

Walther RR, Grossman ME, Troy JL (1981) Basal cell carcinomas on the scalp of a black patient many years after epilation by X-rays, J Dermatol Surg Oncol 7:570–571

Washio H (1969) Retroauricular temporal flap. Plast Reconstr Surg 43:162

White SW, Davis RA, Rodman OG (1980) Surgical management of basal cell carcinoma of the lower lip. J Dermatol Surg Oncol 6:751–754

Zacarian SA (1977) The art and science of cryosurgery. J Dermatol Surg Oncol 3:401–402

Zeller J, Touraine R (1982) Traitement des carcinomes cutanés. Rev Prat 32:2145

Subject Index

MIX
Papier aus verantwortungsvollen Quellen
Paper from responsible sources
FSC® C105338

If you have any concerns about our products,
you can contact us on
ProductSafety@springernature.com

In case Publisher is established outside the EU,
the EU authorized representative is:
Springer Nature Customer Service Center GmbH
Europaplatz 3, 69115 Heidelberg, Germany

Printed by Libri Plureos GmbH
in Hamburg, Germany